Pre Surgical Care

by

Dr. Louis Leonardi

authorHOUSE™

1663 LIBERTY DRIVE, SUITE 200
BLOOMINGTON, INDIANA 47403
(800) 839-8640
WWW.AUTHORHOUSE.COM

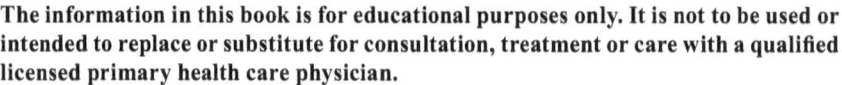

Notice

The information in this book is for educational purposes only. It is not to be used or intended to replace or substitute for consultation, treatment or care with a qualified licensed primary health care physician.

First published by AuthorHouse 9/27/2006

ISBN: 1-4208-5686-3 (sc)
ISBN: 1-4208-6165-4 (dj)

Printed in the United States of America
Bloomington, Indiana

This book is printed on acid-free paper.

While it is impressive to have testimonials from famous authors, celebrities, and prestigious newspapers and magazines we thought it far better to go to the people that could truly evaluate the full depth and overall effectiveness of the Pre Surgical Care book and program ----- the doctors themselves. Here is what they had to say:

"Dr. Leonardi has created a revolutionary book that beautifully bridges the gap between holistic care and medical care. When the necessity of surgery is a fact of life, doesn't it just make sense to be concerned about your physical, emotional, and spiritual well being? Dr. Leonardi's groundbreaking guide will empower you with the exact tools and simple steps to do just that. It's almost hard to imagine why no one has thought to put such a compendium together before."
Dr. Michael Norwood
Arizona

"A brilliant support system for people involved with medical procedures"
Dr. Richard Newman
Alaska

"Very few physicians possess the compassion, understanding, and breadth of awareness and knowledge that Dr. Leonardi is able to share with readers in this remarkable book"
David Schneider, MD
Ohio

"The information and insights in this wonderful book are of a profound nature. And the many true stories make Pre Surgical Care an inspirational and enjoyable book to read."
Dr. Jonathan Spages
New Jersey

"The benefits and value of this book are beyond question for anyone having surgery."
Dr. Katherine Murray
Florida

"A holistic guide for any patient confronting the difficulties of surgery. Dr. Leonardi's years of wisdom, research, and enthusiasm are a contagious remedy that can empower and assist each one of us on our journey of healing"
Dr. Martin Finkelstein
Georgia

Special Incentive
Offer Award

We are offering you a special free healing music CD as a special incentive award to purchase this book or subscribe to our excellent newsletter, which is free, and you can download this inspiring healing music. See the "Special Incentive Offer Award" chapter for all the details.

Table of Contents

Dedicated to

the greatest healers

of all time:

Love

Forgiveness

Peace

Introduction

When I was working in a surgeon's office, I saw a great need for people to prepare themselves more adequately for surgery. Even though they were given handouts to read and follow, even though they were specifically told what to do and what to expect, even though they were told an exact step-by-step procedure, it was just not enough. People would show up and say "I'm here," without realizing the depth of what was actually going to transpire. As a result, they were totally unprepared for the physical trauma, the emotional challenges, and the spiritual shock. They did not realize the depth of what was to happen. They simply needed to be better prepared. They needed to know more and have a better understanding on all levels of body, mind, and spirit.

I was inspired to write this book to support people in being better prepared for invasive procedures. This would optimize conditions to enhance a successful surgery and a more complete recuperation, regeneration, and rejuvenation.

Part I

The Healing Powers of Your Mind

One of the most important parts of this book is Part I. Even though there is specific information on vitamins, minerals, natural herbs, homeopathic medicines, selecting and speaking to your doctor, eliminating anxiety and fear, and more, these opening pages will literally help activate the deepest aspects of your mind's

vast,

incredible,

fantastic,

healing abilities.

Stimulating these healing abilities will help create the best future outcome.

Many times throughout this book, you will read about following the program and becoming an active participant in the preparation for surgery. It may sometimes appear redundant, but this book and program is specifically designed in very, very subtle repetitive ways to scientifically activate your mind to achieve its greatest possible healing powers. Simply reading this book in itself will activate your profound inner healing wisdom. It is specifically designed to stimulate your mind's conscious and subconscious infinite resources to help you heal in all aspects of your mind, body, and spirit.

The mysterious, magical, miraculous healing powers of the mind are far, far beyond anything we have ever imagined. We all have access to these vast healing abilities, and through the pages of this simple book, these incredible healing aspects will be called forth.

This dramatic true story of Jon Zahourek will serve as an interesting example of these little-understood healing powers of the mind. Jon Zahourek is a man who healed himself of a chronic health problem by simply reading a piece of paper.

The Miracle Paper

Jon Zahourek suffered from chronic low back pain. His back pain was from so long ago, he wasn't even sure how it started. Jon's pain was relentless. In his attempt to alleviate his pain he tried everything:

He went to a massage therapist—no help.

He went to a chiropractor—no help

He went to a physical therapist—no help.

He went to an acupuncturist—no help.

He went to a medical doctor—no help.

Jon was resigned to a life of pain. Then, one day when he was working in his studio, something extraordinary happened. He works in an extremely rare and specialized field. Jon is a human anatomical structural artist, clay sculptor. For example, when you go to a museum or when you see a picture in a magazine that shows you the face of a prehistoric man, this face was created from the remains of a partially destroyed, ancient, fossilized human skull. This is the work that Jon Zahourek does. He applies clay sculptured muscles, anatomically correct, layer upon layer, until he completes and reveals the true face of what that person looked like. Depending on what bones he has to begin with, Jon can create not just the face, but any part of the human anatomy.

Though Jon is an expert in his field, he is always developing his skills to his highest degree of excellence. One day, he was working on a model spine, applying the five layers of the muscles of the spine. He would mold and shape each and every muscle in clay, and then apply them to the full-size spine in their exact, correct anatomical position. After working for hours on the anatomical structures, he turned to one of his reference books. As he was reading the book, suddenly something began to happen. He was not sure what it was, but he had a flash, an insight, a new awareness that brought him to a fuller, deeper understanding of exactly how all these individual tissues of bone, cartilages, and muscles came together and created a dynamic human spine.

Jon was thrilled and excited! He jumped up to share with his wife his new revelation. Yet, as he stood up, his mind exploded with an even far more powerful realization—HIS BACK PAIN WAS GONE! After years of persistent problems, he became pain free. Somehow, the greater insight and understanding of the biomechanics of his spine created a shift, a change, a new awareness that freed him from his deep, chronic pain.

Some might say this was simply mind over matter. Others might say it was a coincidence. To Jon Zahourek, it was a miracle.

What you call it doesn't matter. What actually occurred is what is important. Something changed in Jon's mind. Something shifted in Jon's consciousness. With that, something changed in Jon's body*.

This is one of many stories that we have heard throughout all of history about the incredible healing powers of our minds.

None of us has any real idea of the infinity of the healing powers of our minds but we do know that they do exist.

Maybe something in the pages of this book will lead you to your own personal and private "miracle."

Maybe something in this book will give you everything you truly seek:

- o A pain-free body
- o A quiet mind
- o An ease of movement
- o A loving heart
- o A peaceful spirit

---

* This incredible and true story can be downloaded and sent to a friend from our website :http://www.PreSurgicalCare.com.

Mental Techniques

The following mental techniques are very simple and easy to do. They will truly activate the infinite healing powers of your mind.

On a conscious level, you may not be aware of these subtle changes in your body or mind, but be assured that just the same way the television and radio waves are there without your conscious awareness, so too will these mental images produce changes and positive results.

These mental techniques will help activate the unlimited healing powers of your mind. Just give them a try.

Do them every day.

The best time to do them is immediately upon arising and just before going to sleep in the evening.

As an additional benefit, you will also receive a deeper, more nourishing and peaceful sleep.

Take the phone off the hook. Do not be disturbed in any way. Find a quiet place. Make it as peaceful as you can. Sit in a chair or assume the lotus position of sitting on the floor with your legs crossed and your back straight, or lie down on a rug or mat, the bed – anywhere. The most important thing to do is to make yourself comfortable and relaxed.

Affirmations

Affirmations are a way to produce changes in our physiology.

Years of research have demonstrated that the thoughts we think and the words we speak can have a profound effect on our subconscious mind. Consistent positive self-talk can flood over into our conscious mind and create a more powerful state of well-being. This is the power of affirmations.

Close your eyes.

Take three slow, deep breaths, then say each affirmation softly out loud then repeat the process all over again only this time silently in your mind.

"I have a positive mental attitude."
"I have a positive mental attitude."
"I have a positive mental attitude."

"I have a strong, healthy body."
"I have a strong, healthy body."
"I have a strong, healthy body."

"I am calm and tranquil and full of peace."
"I am calm and tranquil and full of peace."
"I am calm and tranquil and full of peace."

Really concentrate on what you are affirming. Sincerely feel the power in your words. Feel free to create a few new positive affirmations of your own. Our thoughts and words make our reality. Take these affirmations into the deepest levels of your spirit and truly believe what you are saying.

These affirmations are available as a free download from our website http://www.PreSurgicalCare.com. They are beautiful calligraphies and suitable for framing. If you email us with your own personal affirmations we will calligraphy them for you free of charge.

Affirmations are great to put all over the house - on doors, on the refrigerator, above the kitchen sink, on the bathroom mirrors. Anywhere. Get creative! Have fun with it!

The Golden White Light Visualization

Close your eyes and imagine a pure, golden white light surrounding your body. Visualize this pure, golden white light penetrating into all the parts of your body.

See it flowing down into your head and neck and down your arms into your fingertips.

Feel it as it gently moves down your chest and into each and every organ.

Visualize this golden white light as it slowly moves down your spine and into your pelvis.

Imagine this golden white light continuing down your legs and into all your muscles. Feel it penetrating all the way into your bones.

Take this golden white light deeply into your feet and out your toes.

Visualize this golden white light flowing deeply into all the cells in your entire body.

Now your body is so full of this golden white light that it radiates all around you.

Visualize it as bright and dazzling as you can.

Hold this image in your mind's eyes for as long as it is comfortable—a few moments or several minutes. Concentrate on this pure, golden white light.

Allow it to become your reality.

Sports Visualization

Years of research studies and massive amounts of experimentation have clearly and definitely proved that mental imaging and visualization can change your physiology. It can alter your heartbeat, blood pressure, respiration, digestive juices, and other systems in your body.

See yourself performing your favorite sports in your mind's eye (tennis, bicycling, running, swimming, etc.) Imagine yourself enjoying these activities.

This will help your body stay physically fit and improve your health.

This is not some casual daydream, but a focused concentration. You must be as exact and specific as possible and use all your senses.

If you are bicycling, do you feel the shoes on your feet? Are you on a mountain trail or pavement? Do you smell the flowers along the trail? Can you hear the wheels as they touch the trail? Do you feel the wind in your hair? Are you surrounded by trees or is it open fields? Do you feel the muscles of the legs pumping? Are you working strong and sweating?

When you do this with single-minded concentration and use all your senses to create a fully detailed and dynamic visualization, your body will experience the physiological changes we mentioned earlier. Your heart will begin to pump faster and harder. Your breathing will become deeper and fuller. Your mind will create these mental images as your body experiences these changes. Some people even begin to sweat!

Just as "real" exercise will help you to be firm and fit, so too will these mental exercises help move you toward maximum health.

Do this exercise every day for at least ten minutes. Play the same sport to perfection or play a new one every day. Have fun!

Being in the Silence

Go into the silence. Begin by taking several slow deep breaths.

Simply make your mind blank and peaceful. Release any wandering thoughts and remain in the deepness of your silence. Do not be concerned if it appears that your mind cannot remain silent. Just focus your concentration on being silent. If you feel that you cannot keep your mind blank, that is fine; just continue to try and stay calm and relaxed.

Do this for a few moments or several minutes.

It's that easy and simple.

Then open your eyes.

Your silent meditation is over[*].

---

[*] The special healing music that is available to you free, is great to listen to while you do these mental techniques. In fact, I listen to it all the time. Go to http://www.PreSurgicalCare.com and read the fascinating true story about how this unique healing music was created.

Part II

The Surgery

The decision has been made.

Alternatives have been tried.

Second and even third opinions have been sought.

Every possibility has been explored.

Maybe you have made this decision out of fear, out of coercion by your family and friends, out of pain, out of hopelessness. It does not make a difference. You have made the decision, therefore only one inevitable conclusion and course of action remains. Let this be the final decision and do not resist it any longer. Let there be

Acceptance

Accept the situation and allow peace in your heart.

The fact is that you have made the decision to have surgery. Now is the time to do everything you can to make it the most calm, peaceful, and successful surgery possible. Yes, there are several definite things you can do to assure yourself that this event will be very successful, but the very first thing that must be done is to accept it and let there be peace in your heart. Until you get through this initial step, there is nowhere else to go. Nothing in this program or any other will be of any benefit until you say "yes" and accept your decision. You are not a victim. Sometimes people think that they are selling out or giving in. They feel guilty or weak or that they are a failure. This is not the case. The final decision to have surgery is yours and yours alone. Let this be a moment of power for you. This is the logical and practical solution to a challenge. Stand in your power and know you have done your best. Know this decision is the most correct one possible because it is **your** decision! This is an important point and it will have a profound effect. You must trust yourself. You must go deep inside and listen to that soft little voice that is now leading you to the most perfect choice. You must know this in your heart of hearts and be at peace with it. It is from this place of knowing that gives you all the strength and power you want to be safe and secure and confident.

By becoming more knowledgeable about the situation and by applying yourself to the *pre surgical care* program, you can:

- Minimize, if not totally eliminate, any negative side effects or complications

- Improve the primary and secondary healing response

- Eliminate allergic reactions

- Quicken repair time

- Minimize over-inflammatory response

- Decrease loss of blood

- Improve cellular tissue regeneration

- Accelerate the entire healing recovery process

- And create many more positive psychological and physiological responses

This can all happen because of a more peaceful and positive state of mind.

This is exactly what *pre surgical care* is about—providing you the educational knowledge to help you become secure, confident, and comfortable about the surgery. It will give you the support you want and need to feel safe and peaceful about this event.

Part I is about activating and stimulating the hidden aspects of your mind's unlimited healing powers.

Part II is about the necessary knowledge to develop and to expand these unlimited healing abilities and to create a positive mental outlook.

Part III is about the vitamins, minerals, herbs, nutrition, and more that will help you produce the desired results we have been speaking about.

After you have accepted the situation and found peace with it, there is another major factor that must be established.

In fact, it is the second most important aspect of this entire chapter (the first being acceptance).

By reading this book and following this program, it will help you to become confident and know you are preparing yourself in a way that is very positive and powerful.

In the same manner that someone must prepare for an athletic event to ensure that they can accomplish their goal, so, too, must we approach surgery. Everyone would agree that if a runner decided to run a marathon, or a musician were to give a concert, certain things must be done. Some preparations must be implemented and followed to ensure the success of the event. In the same way, we must prepare ourselves for surgery—and not just the physical aspects of it. Any runner or musician will tell you the mental and emotional preparations are critically important as well.

This analogy holds true for anyone who will be undergoing surgery. This book and program will be one of the best ways to prepare for this event.

Therefore, please allow me to emphasize the most important aspect of the preparation, the one absolutely essential ingredient necessary to achieve the very best surgical results, the greatest possible approach to ensure the highest results from this book can be written in one word:

Attitude

A true positive attitude supersedes all other conditions. This point cannot be overemphasized.

While Part I activates your mind's vast healing powers and Part II gives you the knowledge, insight, and information of different aspects of the surgery itself (how to select the surgeon, etc.), and Part III gives you exact information that you need on vitamins, minerals, herbs, homeopathic medicines, flower remedies, *it is this positive mental attitude that will give you the greatest beneficial results.*

The most wonderful thing about a positive mental attitude is that it is totally within your control. The story that follows is an allegorical one (as opposed to all the other stories in this book, which are true). It will serve as a powerful example of this point.

The Man of Inspiration

It was hot that day. The heat was intense as it vaporized the water from the men's bodies. The sweat fell like rain, and the smell let every man know that his neighbor wasn't far away. The moans and groans of the men echoed throughout the quarry. Every man was huffing and puffing as they performed their work. It was the complete image of a buzzing hornets' nest.

The foreman at the site was full of compassion and concern for the men. He decided to make a personal inspection to be sure the men were not overburdened by the intensity of the blazing sun in the quarry.

As he descended into the burning fiery pit, all sense of any cooling breeze disappeared. As he descended on each rung of the ladder, hotter and hotter air blasted him from the depths of the stone inferno. "Surely," he thought, "if I continued downward much longer, I'd be at the burning gates of hell."

Luckily, he did not need to go down that far. He reached the rock floor and approached the first man with a question. "What?" responded the first laborer. "How can you ask me how does my work go today? Have you lost all your senses? While you sit up top in the shade of the olive tree, I am suffering down here. Every movement of rock racks my body with pain. My arms and legs grow weary with the toil. Only a fool would allow himself such torture." The man continued to complain and ramble on as the foreman walked away, knowing he would get only negative words of hardship from this man.

He turned to another laborer only a few feet away, again with the same question. The second man replied, "My wife and children and myself appreciate the food my work brings us. It's a good and honest job, and though it's hard and tough, it has made my muscles grow strong and my eyes keen."

Taking another few steps, the foreman addressed the same question to a third laborer. "My day? Look for yourself. Can't you see it!" the third man exclaimed as he lifted his head with a smile on his face. He was filled with enthusiasm and excitement. "Look, I tell you," as he continued to point, "over there will be the vestibule with three beautiful stained glass windows high overhead. There will be the vaulted archway, and over there will be the magnificent doorway. It will be a place for people to come and pray from all of the corners of the empire. It will be the greatest cathedral that man has ever dreamed of. This cathedral will be an inspiration…"

With a gentle nodding of his head, the foreman smiled as he began to ascend the ladder. And even as he climbed, he heard the last man praising the Lord that he was so lucky to place the many stones to create this holy place of grace and glory, this architectural wonder, this magnificent cathedral.

Each of these men was doing exactly the same thing. Each one of them was breaking down rocks, producing bricks, and moving them out of a large quarry and then placing them in the same pile, yet each one of them was leading a completely different life!

If we examine the "objective" physical movements of each man, they looked identical. The rocks were approximately the same size. The weather and environmental conditions were the same. Their foreman was the same and treated them all fairly and equally. In all aspects, they were in the exact same situation, but what appeared the same outside had nothing to do with what was going on inside.

The first man was stuffed with bitterness and anger and complaints, while the second man was thankful and grateful. The third laborer was filled with vision and awe and passion and purpose and meaning.

Three men…

Three different lives…

Which one are you?

It's simply a matter of choice!

It's simply a matter of attitude!

Hopefully, you are the third person who is learning how to see everything in a positive light, who is full of energy, a person who is using this event to create a more purposeful and meaningful life, a person using these circumstances to act as a catalyst for a better future full of appreciation and gratitude and happiness.

It's your decision.

It's a matter of

perception,

choice,

attitude.

Let there be peace in your heart!

The Surgeon

With the acceptance of the surgery and a positive mental attitude firmly established, the relationship with the surgeon is the next most important issue. *Not the surgeon himself, but the relationship between the two of you.*

Most people think that the skill of the surgeon is the most important factor. This is not true! It is the relationship between you and the surgeon that will yield the best positive results.

To begin with, forget all the facts, statistics, generalities, politics, and clichés you have heard before about doctors. Put aside all the jokes you've heard about surgeons and golf and any other negative things. You are about to enter into a relationship with a concerned, feeling, caring human being.

Your relationship with your surgeon is one of the most important relationships you will ever have with another person. In many ways, your very life may depend on it. It is not one to fall into casually. Consider this, no matter how good a surgeon is…

his skill,

his experiences,

his accolades,

his reputation—

they mean nothing, absolutely nothing, unless you and he establish a warm, caring human bond—not a dependency or emotional attachment, but a relationship based on mutual respect, sincerity, integrity, honesty, and truthfulness. These are some of the most essential factors involved with establishing a safe, efficient, and successful surgery. Create a relationship with the surgeon that will accomplish this goal. If you feel like a number lost in a vast maze or a *persona non grata,* you should not have the doctor as your surgeon. Speak to your doctor and express your fears and concerns. Maybe he can help bring you through any of these negative feelings and continue to reinforce your positive mental attitude and even take it to a higher level.

To illustrate this point, please allow me to speak to you about a very personal experience I had once, to indicate the depth of subtleties that exist when two people come together. For many years, this occurrence baffled me, and even to his day, I am not sure what transpired. It happened about ten years ago.

The Lady of Mystery

I met a lady one day. I was immediately attracted to her and she to me. We were both delighted. It appeared to both of us that we liked each other very much. We began to date, and after a short time, we began to live together. We were very happy together and had fun times. We never argued. We were enjoying each other's company immensely, but we soon came to realize that it would be a short-term relationship. We were different in our paths, goals, and dreams. In the long run, we knew it would not work out. As an example, I love to travel. I had a great desire to explore the world. I wanted to experience this incredible planet. Diane, on the other hand, had no interest whatsoever in traveling. She was very happy and content in staying home, and did not want to go anywhere. Anyone can clearly see that this was an incompatibility of interests.

There was no right or wrong here or good or bad. It was what it was, and we both accepted it. We spoke about it and decided to stay together and continue onwards until we felt it was time to move on separately. After about six wonderful, joyous months together, it became apparent that it was time to split up. This was all done very amicably with many hugs and kisses. While we shared in our sorrows and grief, there was a great deal of sincere emotion between us; there was no anger or bitterness or hostility or anything like that. We just said goodbye.

To understand the point of this short drama and its relationship to you and your surgeon, we must digress for a moment and turn to something completely unrelated—my driving activities.

For those of you who have read my biography in the back of the book, you know that I was a New York City taxicab driver. I did this for two interesting years. (Yes, it was very interesting, but that's a whole different book.) In addition to this, I drove cross-country several times, drove a motorcycle up and down the East Coast, and also drove a monster dump truck as a summer job as a young college student. So when I met Diane, not only was I a seasoned driver with twenty years of experience, I was a professional driver. When you drive a taxi in New York City for two years, you qualify as an expert. Through all those years, I had an impeccable driving record. I never even had a fender-bender or a car scratch. This in itself was nothing spectacular but there was one very short, precise period in time when I did have not one but several accidents. I hit two garbage pails each at different times. I also hit three birds, each at different times. I crashed into a large oil barrel with a blinking light on it that you would see on the side of the highway. I ran over a raccoon once and I was even run off the road. All this happened at one very small, exact period in time—the six months that I was with Diane and only during the six months I was with Diane—nothing before or after. She was in the car only twice on all these occurrences. It was the same car, the same roads, the same everything. As far as I could tell, I drove the same as I always did. This appeared and still does seem very strange to me, but it did happen. How did this transpire? My only answer was that there was something in our relationship that did not blend together properly.

As I said earlier, it was all a mystery to me until one day a few years later, I was given a possible clue. I saw Diane at a restaurant. She was on a lunch break and I joined her. It was very nice to see her and we had a pleasant lunch together. In the course of the conversation, she made a comment, quite innocently and casually. It was something she had never expressed to me before. She said that she resented that I was such a great driver. I always drove when we were together, regardless of whose car it was. She herself felt she was a very poor driver. She had a low self-esteem of her driving abilities. In her eyes, I was always relaxed and comfortable behind the wheel whereas she was always a "nervous wreck" (her words). Did these hidden feelings of resentment and anger and jealousy have anything to do with those six months of my driving accidents? Was there something in her mind, something in her psyche that attacked my mind? Was there something that altered my judgments in the split moment that the decisions demanded to be made? Did I render different decisions than I normally would have? Was my mind impaired somehow in some subtle way and lost in the vast unknown?

I do not know. I have no conscious awareness of it, but what about our subconscious mind? Does it have some way to connect with these most subtle of thoughts? What is it that creates these things we call thoughts, these impulses that seemingly arise from nowhere, these ideas that suddenly appear in our minds?

Like the man who, on his way to work, decided to stop and buy donuts for everyone at the office, so he arrived late to work.

Or the other man who bought a new pair of shoes a few days before, and on his way to the office, felt so uncomfortable in them that he decided, in that very moment, to return them, so he arrived late to work.

And then there was another man who looked at his daughter as she prepared to go to school and thought, "I have not been with my girl enough lately. Why not take her to school today on my way to work." This is something he had not done in a long time but somehow, in some way, this innocent thought came to him on this particular day at this particular time, so he took her to school, and as a result he was late to the office that day.

To these three men, it was just another ordinary day, or so it seemed ….

These are all true stories. Again, I ask you where do these seemingly insignificant thoughts come from that change our lives—forever?

What do these three stories share in common? All three men worked on the 86th floor of the World Trade Center and were not there on 9/11 because they followed these inner feelings, these fleeting impulses, these spontaneous thoughts.

Please read this book with full concentration. Embrace this book on a far deeper level than it superficially appears.

Take it to the deepest aspects of your mind.

In some way, your mind and your surgeon's mind have become united together. Be as certain as you can be that this surgeon and this relationship is the best that it can be[*].

Now that you are sure, be grateful. Appreciate it. Give thanks.

---

[*] If you have not selected a surgeon yet we have set up a referral program to assist you in finding one in your area.

To further your relationship with your doctor, speak to him about your fears and concerns.

Ask him your questions.

1. How long before my *complete* recovery?
2. Will I need to be on drugs and medications after the surgery?
3. How long will I be out of work?
4. Will I be in pain?
5. Will I be incapacitated in any way?
6. Do I need to make any changes, for example, will I be bedridden after surgery, or will I require in-home assistance?
7. Is he knowledgeable in nutrition?
8. Will there be a scar and what will it look like?
9. Has he considered my personal sensitivities?
10. Will I need another surgery in the future or is this permanent?

Assume nothing. Ask all your myriad of questions.

Ask him about his belief in "miracles." While they may be rare, is such a thing possible? Has he ever heard a "miracle" story from any of his colleagues? Does he think that the body's abilities to heal itself are truly amazing and marvelous?

If it's important to you, ask him if he believes in prayer? Does he believe in God? As a patient and as a person, you have a right to ask these meaningful questions and any other questions you may have, and get answers that set you to rest and peace.

Go over every part of the procedure. This will help alleviate your fears and anxieties. Make sure he answers all your questions to your satisfaction. Do not be hurried or harried by his manner. If he does not give you his time to answer your questions, what makes you think he will slow down enough when you are in the surgery with him? Take your time. Be polite, but ask your questions and get your answers to your satisfaction.

Be steadfast—do not be pressured or rushed along. The surgeon works for you and with you—together, you are a team. See it that way, communicate that vision with him. He is not your boss—you work together. Do not be intimidated!

Be diplomatic, but be direct.

Be thankful, and let him know how much you appreciate his giving you his valuable time and skill.

Another fact that should be considered: *Under no circumstances will you allow anyone else to perform this surgery.* Accept no last-minute changes or emergency changes or change of doctor. Simply make another appointment for your surgery. In most circumstances, this may be a moot point but speak to your doctor and obtain his promise on this at the beginning of your relationship and again a few days before the event.

Be cheerful and friendly. The doctor is a person, too. Your doctor is a sincere and caring individual. He has dedicated years of his life to serving people just like you through severe traumas and trying times. Do not be swayed by media hype and the very few who have been involved in scams or scandals. Do not be influenced or confused by the politics and flaws of the organizations. We are speaking of a real, feeling, loving human being. Over the last few years, doctors have been maligned and abused. It has become commonplace, politically correct, and socially acceptable to bash medical doctors. Please do not follow these unjustified and unreasonable judgments. Make your own unbiased, personal assessment of your doctor.

You are working with an individual person who needs your help and cooperation and kindness, just as you want and need his. The more you give to him, the more he will give to you. The vast majority of doctors are good, honest, trustworthy, compassionate people under a great deal of pressure. They are people using all their skills and talents and experience to help you. Who cannot marvel at the surgeon who can restore sight, remove a painful abscessed tooth, replace a finger, help the lame to walk, repair a damaged face, remove a brain tumor, open clogged arteries, replace an organ, eliminate a cancer...?

These are truly wondrous and awesome abilities, and now your surgeon is using all his abilities to help YOU. Be thankful. You must know that he is doing his very best for you and doing everything he can for you. This must be your truth. If you doubt it, if you question it, if you don't know it, then either find a new surgeon fast, or have a more intimate conversation and communication with the one you have now. You must become completely at peace and calm with your doctor. Your full trust, belief, and confidence in your doctor will make a tremendous impact on the results.

Any hidden resentments and hostilities towards your doctor will have some negative effects—no matter how subtle—on some level. Think back to the story of "The Lady of Mystery." By having feelings of sincerity and trust in your doctor's integrity, it will assist him so he can perform to his highest ability. This will create a "win-win" situation for everyone. Affirm and accept the doctor to your utmost, and as a team, the greatest success will be achieved. It is in these ways that you will inspire your surgeon to give you his absolute best.

Some of you may consider these glowing portraits of praise the words of a biased, ingratiating surgeon speaking about friends, peers, and colleagues. Nothing could be further from the truth. The author of this book, Dr. Louis Leonardi, holds degrees as a Doctor of Chiropractic, Doctor of Naturopathy, and Doctor of Homeopathy. In his intense desire for knowledge in the healing arts, he has traveled and studied all over the world. He has worked with the shamans in the hidden rainforests of South America, and the medicine men in the wild jungles of Africa. He has also studied with the ancient ayurvedic healers of India, and the legendary acupuncturists of Asia.

He thinks of himself, more than anything else, as a Doctor of Holistic Medicine. As a result, he has spent a lifetime telling people not to go to surgeons, not to take drugs, not to undergo harsh, invasive therapies, but instead to seek alternatives! He believes in informing people about alternatives like chiropractic care, acupuncture, and homeopathy. He speaks to people about dietary and nutritional changes, and he encourages them to seek natural, herbal remedies as possible substitutes for prescription medication.

The consideration has been to begin with a simpler, more conservative approach. But when these more gentle and conservative ways are not effective, then by all means, turn to the greatness of surgery. For when surgery is necessary, this is the key word—*necessary*—it is indeed amazing. Surgery should not be the first resort! The question is one of degree, and when all other approaches and conservative treatments have been unsuccessful, then, as a last resort, surgery should be employed. Appreciate it. Be thankful for it. Applied in this manner, it is indeed truly marvelous and fantastic.

Part III

The Practical Application

One Month Before

This is a highly successful, achievable program. It is easy to follow and will give you great results, but you must *do* the program to receive these positive results. A program is only as good as how it is followed. Results can only come about by action.

By reading Parts I and II, you have already received subtle new cues and insights, and a better understanding to approach this event.

Simply reading this book

fully,
    slowly,
        carefully,
            completely

will help you activate your vast healing abilities and create more of your own "infinite healing power."

Now that Part I has activated your mind to its highest level of healing, and Part II has helped you achieve a positive mental attitude, Part III will continue to give you more specific information on what will assist you in preparing for your surgery on all levels of your body, mind, emotions, and spirit.

Use common sense when following these recommendations. Be sure to follow your doctor's advice first and foremost throughout this entire program. There are many suggestions and steps that will help you prepare you for this event, but you need not do every single one. If you can, that's fine, but if not, that's fine, too. It is far more important to stay stress-free and relaxed. Do the best you can. By reading this book, you are already demonstrating your desire and willingness to become more involved in your healing. This commitment alone will give you a better degree of self-confidence and security. Through your increased knowledge, you will be able to stay more calm and peaceful.

DIET

There is no "special diet" for surgery. The food we eat always has a profound effect on our health, but now is not the proper time to make any major dietary changes. You do not want to produce any tension or stress by trying to start some new special diet, but there are some very valuable suggestions and recommendations that you can follow:

Drink spring or distilled water, not tap water, unless it is purified in some way.

Increase your water intake to a minimum of four glasses a day.

Reduce or avoid as much as possible:

> *sugar*
> *soft drinks*
> *white flour*
> *desserts*
> *fried food*
> *caffeine*
> *alcohol*
> *smoking*

In relation to what you do eat, try to obtain the highest quality food you can. If you eat eggs, purchase organic eggs. If you want chicken, buy 'free range' chicken. If you want chocolate, get real, pure chocolate. Ice cream? Purchase an ice cream without preservatives or other types of artificial ingredients. Obtain fresh fruits and vegetables that have been grown organically - without the use of herbicides, pesticides, or other toxic chemicals. You can even find organic wines and beers. Your local health food store will have most of these items or information about them. You can also go to our newsletter and read about a dynamic new movement that's happening in the health food market, which is making food shopping interesting, entertaining, and fun.

That's it! It's that simple. Just make these easy changes—all or some—do the best you can. It is your choice. If you feel pressure at trying to reduce your caffeine intake or skip your dessert, then let go, have it, and enjoy it. These are merely suggestions. They will be very helpful and effective if followed, but it is more important to stay centered and balanced as much as possible. As stated several times throughout this book, the preeminent consideration is to remain relaxed and maintain a positive mental attitude. It will have a powerful beneficial effect on your healing and regeneration.

FRESH JUICING

We have included this section on fresh juicing for those who have juicers and are already familiar with making fresh, raw juices. If you are not familiar with juicing, please move on to the next chapter*.

While rewards of fresh fruit and vegetable juices are extremely well-documented and established, it is not our intent to overload you with new "stuff." If juicing is already part of your lifestyle now, here are some ideas for specific juices. There are no "wrong" choices, so do not be overly concerned about the selection. Any of these juices will have a very positive healing effect on your body. These basic recommendations are for the main constitutional systems involved in the surgery:

Blood (heart, arteries, etc.): beets, wheat grass
Nerves: potatoes, nectarines
Endocrine (reproductive organs, adrenals, thyroid, pituitary, etc.): artichokes, wheat grass, spinach
Musculoskeletal (joints, muscles, bones): greens
Immune system: parsley, lemon (in very small amounts)
Digestion: cabbage, papaya
Respiration: greens
Urinary: (kidneys, bladder): watermelon *(by itself—not with carrot juice)*

---

* Ever had a freshly prepared fruit juice or carrot juice or mixed vegetable juice? Many local health food stores can provide this service for you. Try it, you may like it.

Lymphatic: apple, wheat grass

Remember, all juices are mixed with ¾ or more of carrot juice.

A *very small* amount of ginger or garlic or lemon can be used in any of these juices. Let your taste be your guide. If it is too strong, add more carrot juice or reduce the other food(s). An apple can be used sometimes to add sweetness, but *never use sugar or honey.* Play with the juices. Try different combinations. Have fun. The most important thing is that it tastes good. Enjoy!

Drink a glass every morning. It's a great way to begin the day. Continue with fresh juicing for not only a month after the surgery, but consider it as a regular lifestyle!

EXERCISE

Images of powerful muscles, sweating bodies, and intense competitions are the usual internal response to the word "exercise." However, this is far from what we are suggesting. What we do suggest is walking in the park and spending some time relaxing with the trees and the flowers. This would be a wonderful benefit to you. Of course, if you cannot walk or do any type of physical activities for any reason, then return to the sports visualization. This will be of great benefit to you. Remember, you are preparing yourself for surgery, and walking every day will help tone your muscles, improve your circulation, and increase your organs' functions to their optimal levels. *This is essential.*

Maybe walking outdoors is a question of time. You do not have enough time to go for a walk in the park or go for a swim or ride a bicycle or "something" physical. If you really examine this from a different perspective, maybe, just maybe, it's a matter of commitment. Perhaps it's this "lack of time" that has helped produce more stress and tension that has added to this problem. If you think you have a "good" reason or excuse for not having the time to go for a walk in the park, let me tell you about my inspiring friend, Bob Wieland.

The Legend of Bob Wieland

He seemed like any ordinary guy with an ordinary dream—he wanted to run in the New York City Marathon. While in itself, the desire to prepare, to compete, to finish a marathon is not usually considered "fantastic" or "extraordinary," in this particular case, it was more like "mission impossible."

One day, Bob decided it was time to take full action and pursue his goal of running the New York City Marathon. He began to get in shape and train for this grueling twenty-six-mile event. He figured it would take him about a year before he could be ready. So he made a plan, checked the date, set the goal, and took action:

He practiced five days a week.
He began a weight training program.
He prepared mentally every day for the challenge.

Finally, the day arrived. He had his numbers pinned on the front and back of his T-shirt, and with 25,000 runners, he eagerly awaited the start of the race. Bob was lost in the pack. He was there, though, and he was ready to go, but more importantly, he was determined to finish. He had come this far, after all the training, all the sweat, all the preparation…he was absolutely determined to complete the marathon.

51

The traditional gun signaled the start of the race. Because of the large number of runners, it was a full forty-five minutes before Bob got to the starting line. He didn't think much about it. He didn't use a watch. He didn't care what his time was or anything like that. He had only one dedicated, unwavering, committed goal: he was going to finish the New York City Marathon.

After about two hours and ten minutes, the leaders started coming across the finish line. The roar of the crowd, the flash of cameras, and the gala hoopla was a splendid finale to a race well run, but Bob was moving along at his own pace—slow and steady. Runner after runner passed him by. There were a few scattered here and there alongside the course who stopped and tended their wounds, their hurts, their pains— either physical or psychological. Some caught Bob's eyes as he nodded and acknowledged their bravery and willingness to participate in the race. The hours continued to tick on.

Eventually, Bob was all alone. But Bob kept on going. Twilight came, and as the sun set and the moon rose, Bob gave a prayer of thanks. He continued throughout the night, taking short, random breaks to relax and rest.

As the sun rose the next day, Bob was still out there continuing the course. As he went from borough to borough (the course goes through each of the five boroughs that make up New York City), the sun went down for the second day. Slowly and steadily, Bob continued on. He didn't notice the pain or the stress or the exhaustion. It was just part of accepting the challenges of the race. Bob knew these challenges would be involved in completing his goal. He was making progress, and every moment, he was coming closer to the finish line.

The sun rose again on the third day, and it was a happy day for Bob, because today he knew he would cross the finish line. Sure enough, hours later, under the blistering hot sun, Bob entered Central Park toward the finish line of the race. Someone saw Bob with his number on and was amazed.

"Impossible!" he thought. "The marathon finished days ago! This guy couldn't have been out there all this time. No way!"

His curiosity and interest and awe of the intense, unimaginable, and incredible scene he was witnessing prompted him to approach Bob and run alongside him. Actually, he needed only to walk to keep up with Bob. Bob just kept on moving slowly and steadily.

"The race is over! It ended three days ago!" he addressed Bob.

"Not for me," Bob replied. "The race isn't over until I cross the finish line."

"But the officials, the people, everyone is gone."

"That's OK."

"But the finish line is down, the shoots, everything is gone. No one, nothing is left, nothing."

"Lucky for me I memorized the course, or I would have gotten lost!" Bob laughed.

"But you're last."

Bob just kept on.

"I'm sorry to tell you, you are *really last*."

Suddenly, Bob saw the finish line. The finish line? It was just a small line, a white line on a piece of cement. The emotions that were created by that white line were beyond explanation. Some people's entire lives revolved around that thin, white line. It was a symbol for every human emotion you could imagine:

glory,
>pride,
>>failure,
>>>gratitude,
>>>>happiness,
>>>>>disappointment,
>>>>>>agony,
>>>>>>>ecstasy!!!

Yet, in itself, it was nothing except a small, simple, plain white line.

"Sorry, guy, but you are really out of it. You are dead last. In fact, you probably hold the record for being the last of the last in the New York City Marathon."

Undaunted by the stranger's unsupportive, negative attitude, Bob crossed the finish line.

He paused, he stopped, he rested.

Looking up at the friendly stranger, Bob said, "Last?"

"Oh, yeah man, like last."

"Last?"

"Real last."

"If you ask me," Bob said smiling, "I could never be last."

"Well you are."

"If you ask me, I could never be last. If you ask me," Bob asserted, "I finished ahead of 200 million people who never even entered the race!"

The man was stunned. He was emotionally moved by Bob's truthful words. He could do or say nothing more. Bob continued on his merry way.

Bob was

elated,

euphoric,

ecstatic.

He was thrilled beyond words. He had achieved his goal and fulfilled his commitment.

You may be wondering why it took Bob three full days to run a marathon. If he were in a wheelchair, he could have finished in a few hours. Crutches? No way. Oh, did I forget to mention *Bob Wieland has no legs! He did the entire marathon on his hands.*

This true story is about exercise on the surface, but it's far more meaningful than that. One can easily see that it is about attitude. And it is in this attitude that the most noble and virtuous qualities of the human spirit spring forth. Qualities like:

courage,

determination,

persistence,

commitment,

vision,

excellence.

Is this current challenge bringing out the best in you?

VITAMINS

Before we can address the important role of vitamins and minerals in the *pre surgical care program,* we must understand what the recommended daily allowances (RDA) are and why they not very useful for us.

Recommended daily allowances for all vitamins and minerals were established to keep a person from getting ill or developing a disease. This means they are the very minimal amounts necessary for people to keep them from getting sick. They are not designated to put anyone in a condition of optimal health. Anyone can clearly see, with this understanding, the necessity of superseding these recommendations. First we must help create higher levels of optimal health and then beyond that to handle the greater emotional stress and physical trauma of the event.

A surgery is far beyond the "normal" circumstances we encounter on a daily basis. Our bodies will require much more than the usual amounts of vitamins and minerals on this fact alone. To ensure a fast, quick, and complete recovery, it would behoove us to take larger amounts of these supplements to prepare ourselves for the greater demands that are being placed upon us because of this event.

With this in mind, it would appear obvious to support ourselves in the best ways possible, hence the taking of these very critical vitamins and minerals in higher dosages. This will allow us to achieve our goals of moving us into a state of optimal health and to prepare us for a rapid and complete recuperation and recovery.

We have also considered any toxicity effects from the larger dosages. Even though they are double, triple, quadruple or more of the "normal" amount, no toxic side effects have been known. Therefore, these higher dosages, within these ranges, are totally safe.

If this program is being used for a child, these recommendations must be modified.

Always seek the advice and guidance of your doctor throughout this entire program.

There is one vitamin that your body does not produce. There is one vitamin that has been researched and utilized for over forty years with great safety and success. There is one vitamin that has been involved with all aspects of the healing process, from the deepest levels of biological cellular repair to the highest levels of tissue regeneration.

While, at times, it was the center of hot debate and controversy, one factor always remained constant—its recognition and acknowledgment as the number one vitamin in the healing process. *That vitamin is vitamin C!*

Yes, there are many vitamins that can be recommended, but this program is not about recommending vitamin therapy. *Pre surgical care* is about making sure you are optimally prepared and supported for this particular impending future event. The use of vitamin C will help establish this condition.

The biggest question now that needs an answer is not as much "what" to take, but "how much" to take. All previous guidelines for vitamins and minerals that have been scientifically established are not applicable now and cannot be employed because these guidelines exist for normal day-to-day life.

Any invasive procedure into the body is far removed from our daily activities and would command larger-than-usual doses of supplementation. With this understanding as a reference tool, it is suggested that you slowly increase the normal recommended dosage of vitamin C until it is tripled or even quadrupled.

If, in the process of increasing to this higher amount of vitamin C, any unusual or different symptoms appear (some but certainly not all) like gas or bloating or diarrhea or just anything new that shows up, stop for a day and then reduce the amount until all the symptoms cease and your body is functioning normally again. Once this amount is comfortably established, stay on it the entire month (except the day before, the day of surgery, and the day after) and continue on it for the month after.

The next most important vitamins in relation to the entire healing process are vitamins A and E. These two vitamins are good for many aspects of the healing process, especially for cuts and tears, either internally on your fascia or externally on your skin. Along with zinc (more on zinc in the mineral section) these three substances form a dynamic, synergistic interaction that supports and allows their full absorption and usage in the regeneration of the tissue changes caused by the surgery. But this is just the beginning of their benefits.

Vitamin A has been shown to be a highly successful booster to the immune system. This is the system that protects us from a multitude of potential problems, especially infections. It insures the plentiful reproduction of immune cells that line the airways and digestive tracts. This forms a potent line of defense against infections and many other possible complications.

Since our bodies cannot synthesize vitamin A without its precursor, it must be absorbed from the foods we eat. Under normal circumstances, there are usually adequate amounts of vitamin A in our diets, but as indicated before, these are not normal conditions. The inclusion of vitamin A in the *pre surgical care* program will help immensely.

According to the recommended daily allowances, the suggested dosage for vitamin A is 2,500 international units (IUs) per day. As stated in the beginning of this chapter, the recommended daily allowances are the minimum dosages to ward off sickness and disease—not to put us in a state of optimal health. With this understanding firmly established and vitamin A's long-standing nontoxic record, we suggest 20,000 IUs of vitamin A per day. This will give you all you need to prepare for this event and keep your body at optimum health.

Vitamin E has emerged as another superstar in the nutritional world. One reason is because it has been associated with many beneficial results for a wide variety of biological functions. Some of these successful biological activities are as an antioxidant, an anti-inflammatory, a defense against cardiovascular disease, and even cancer. Vitamin E is also well-known as a promoter for skin healing. It is known to make scar tissue more elastic and flexible, both internally and externally. These are important points to consider. Vitamin E works on a deep cellular level. It is a powerful enhancer for the metabolic system, and its booster effect to the immune system places vitamin E as a prime supplement in the *pre surgical care* program.

The recommended daily allowance for vitamin E is about 10 IUs per day, but the recommended dosage by most experts, because of its well-known healing aspects, is usually about 400-800 IUs per day. Some researchers go as high as 40,000 IUs per day with no known side effects, but we agree with the nutritional experts and suggest 400-800 IUs per day[*].

We reiterate that the range we suggest is an excellent amount to prepare you for surgery and in maintaining your body in a state of optimal health.

Please take special note here to inform your doctor of any supplements that you are taking, not only in relation to

---

[*] Some research has indicated that vitamin E may produce thinning of the blood. If there is any possibility that this may be a concern for your particular type of surgery then it is imperative to stop taking vitamin E two weeks before the surgery and be sure to speak to your doctor on this point!

this program but in all aspects of your nutritional supplementation.

MINERALS

The minerals in your body are the building blocks, the very foundation that your body is composed of. Mineral balance in your body is essential. They are the co-enzymes and catalysts that are needed for almost every biochemical reaction that occurs in your body.

Scientists have identified some sixty to seventy minerals to date, but some scientists think that the body is composed of every element on the planet.

The minerals are divided into two major categories: macro minerals (calcium, chloride, magnesium, phosphorus, potassium, sodium, sulfur) which are usually thought of in terms of grams and milligrams; and micro minerals (all the remaining minerals) usually thought of in terms of micrograms, millionths of a gram, or even less.

The size of the mineral is not important. What is important is that all the minerals in your body are in the proper amount and in the proper balance. To have all the minerals in your body and reliably accessible is absolutely essential.

Besides being the building blocks in your body, they are also the major catalysts. Without the proper catalysts, the biochemical reactions cannot occur. In many instances, unless the minerals are there, the vitamins themselves are totally useless. This can lead to pathological processes and diseases.

Since our bodies are performing billions of biochemical reactions every moment, you can clearly see how a full supply of minerals is absolutely necessary. This will allow the body to function and perform at its highest level.

Luckily, this can be easily accomplished by taking a multi-mineral formula.

The following is a true personal and humorous story about how I came to know about the true necessity of minerals in our bodies.

A Casual Visit

It was just a casual visit to my friend Steven Halpern's house, but it became something more. Sometime during the visit, I was in the kitchen, and I saw a small bottle with a label on it. I was curious and picked it up to examine it more closely. It was a small bottle of multi-mineral liquid concentrate. "Wow!" I was impressed. It had almost every mineral known to man in it, (several which I never heard of) taken from a pure, safe, natural source. More importantly, it was a balanced combination in a form I knew to be readily absorbable by the body.

Dr. Halpern (Ph.D.) is usually well-informed on nutritional matters, and my interest was certainly stimulated, so I thought I'd give it a try. As I opened the dropper spout and lifted the bottle up over my head, I called out to Steven in the next room, asking him if I could try some of this "trace mineral formula"

Steven's immediate response was "Yes." Since I knew Steven's generous nature, I knew he would not begrudge me a few drops of this multi-mineral formula, so I had already assumed the necessary position. I merely tipped the bottle over a little more, and a few drops fell directly into my mouth. Simultaneously, as the drops touched my tongue, I heard him continue to say, "Be sure to put it in some juice first. It's very concentrated and powerful and should be diluted or it will really sting. There's juice in the refrigerator."

"Ahhhhhoooooooooowwwwww..." It was too late—the deed was done. Hearing my anguished howl, he rushed in, instantly perceiving the entire scenario. He let out a whopping laugh. He knew the "liquid mineral formula" would not hurt me, but that a direct application on the tongue, such as I had done, would have an *intense sting*.

As you may know, it is extremely rare to take a vitamin or mineral and feel an *immediate* change. It takes weeks or longer for most supplements to really affect and improve your energy levels. Not this time!

What happened at this point was fantastic, and to this very day, I can recall it so vividly. The instant the "liquid mineral formula" drops touched my tongue, it was like being splashed by a refreshing palm beach summer wave. It was like a euphoric surge of power. I felt a wonderful sense of energy and well-being about me.

Now I was more than impressed—I was committed. I viewed this small, plain bottle in my hand as if it were an elixir of transformation. I was overcome with a feeling of invincibility. I just stood there staring at Steven with my jaw dropped wide open. Still laughing, he opened the refrigerator and poured me a glass of cranberry juice (excellent for the kidneys) and handed it to me.

It took me a few moments to respond, but eventually I reached out and took the glass from his hand. After taking a quick sip, I joined him in his laughter, and laugh we did, as he shared with me that he had had the same experience! With his comments, we both knew exactly what happened to each other, and we just laughed and laughed and laughed!

One of the reasons I share this story with you is because I had no idea that I could have been mineral deficient and I never would have realized this without an experience like this.

Again, I tell you this personal story to provide an example of how important it is to make sure you have all the necessary minerals in your body.

As for individual minerals, there is one mineral that outshines all the others in relationship to healing. It has a long, thoroughly researched, safe, and effective history. It is known as the *healing* mineral. That mineral is zinc.

Like vitamin A, zinc cannot be produced in our bodies. Zinc is needed by every cell in the body. It is involved with millions of biochemical reactions every moment. Without zinc as the catalyst in our bodies, none of these reactions can occur.

Zinc is necessary for a wide range of beneficial results. It fights colds and flu, affects many of the hormones, promotes the repair of skin tissue, keeps hair healthy, stops infections, and heals cuts and wounds. This is only a few of zinc's impressive list of healing properties and because of it, zinc will be very beneficial to you now.

Another mineral associated with accelerating the healing process, especially of connective tissue (muscles, ligaments, fascia, etc.) is manganese.

Manganese is known to be very useful in healing cuts and wounds. These two minerals plus the other recommendation in the *pre surgical care* program will continue to build a better body and prepare you for this impending operation.

Take 100 mg of zinc daily. This appears to be the body's upper limit for full absorption. Do not take more. It will not have any toxic side effects, but larger dosages are not necessary.

Take 20 mg of manganese daily. This will be an excellent amount for healing the connective tissue.

HERBS

Somewhere, lost in the antiquity of history, are the origins of our finest medicines to help heal and cure the body—*herbs*. After many centuries of use, herbs have become more and more refined and perfected. In today's modern world, through the folklore and wisdom of the ages, to the vast information gained from clinical studies, combined with the latest technological scientific research, herbs have achieved their highest use of efficiency and effectiveness. In fact, almost every single pharmaceutical drug on the market today is based on an *"active ingredient"* found in herbs. It would be very beneficial to use these potent, natural remedies to help create optimum conditions in preparation for surgery.

Following this idea, here are some simple guidelines to select the finest quality of herbs. The exact herbs themselves are given at the end of the chapter.

1. Get *real* herbs, not active ingredients.
2. Read the label to ensure that it is organic or wild crafted. If it doesn't state this explicitly, then you can be sure it is not organic or wild crafted.

---

* Please note that nothing from the outside can heal or cure the body. Only the power, the energy, the force, the life *within the body* can heal and cure it. Anything from the outside can only help the body heal itself.

3.   Read the label closely and be sure it is what you are looking for and not full of fillers, diversifiers, and powders.
4.   Do not be fooled by the use of the word "natural." This word is non-regulatory and can be extremely (intentionally) misleading.
5.   For internal usage, herbal tinctures are usually far superior to tablets, which are usually better than capsules. This is generally true, but not always.

As a final note, some herbs are multi-functional and can be added and used at any time. As an example, garlic, goldenseal, and echinacea are some of the best antibiotics known to man, and they are completely natural, gentle, safe, and effective to use.

While there are hundreds and hundreds of herbs to choose from, the selection can be narrowed down very easily and safely and effectively by using the "constitutional" approach. This method uses the herbs necessary for the complete overall major system involved with this event. As an example, any knee or shoulder surgery must involve the musculoskeletal system. Another example would be heart surgery. This would involve the arterial system of the body. By using the "constitutional" method, you can select those particular herbs needed to be used for the major system involved. The following "constitutional" chart gives you the appropriate herbs to select.

Select the constitutional herbs from the following chart for your involved system:

System	Recommended Herb
Endocrine Glands (hormonal)	Wild yam, Licorice, Ginseng
Immune system	Golden Seal, Garlic, Mistletoe
Digestive system	Aloe Vera, Barberry, Fennel, Peppermint, Mugwart, Spearmint
Musculoskeletal system	Comfrey, Ginger, Calendula, Arnica
Blood (arterial) system	Echinacea, Milk Thistle, Lily of the Valley, Hawthorne
Lymphatic system	Cascada Sagrada, Cleavers Herb
Nervous system	Skull Cap, St. John's Wort, Valerian Root Chamomile, Blue Vervain, Cola Nut
Respiratory system	Mullin, Chaparral, Goldenrod
Reproductive system	Ginseng, Saw Palmetto, Helonias root
Urinary system	Juniper Berry, Yarrow Flower, Buchu Leaves

Select only one or two herbs as close as possible for the system involved with your surgery. For instance, if it is a ligament tear, the musculoskeletal system would be involved; if an organ, the digestive system; if an infection or cancer, it would involve the immune system.

If you're currently taking herbs, then take double the recommended dosage of the constitutional herbs that you have selected. If you do not usually take herbs, then the recommended dosage will be very effective.

Add Lobelia to any of the constitutional herbs you select, because Lobelia acts as an herbal enhancer and will boost the power of all of these herbs.

Be assured that it would be rare, if not impossible, to select a bad or wrong herb, as they are all multifaceted and wide-ranging in their marvelous healing abilities. The simple addition of these constitutional master herbs will enhance your well-being immensely[*].

---

[*] You may be interested in herbs that can help with specific health problems or enhance prescription medications. Through our free newsletter you can obtain information like this. You can even become a "Certified Master Herbalist". Go to http://www.PreSurgicalCare.com to find out how.

HOMEOPATHIC MEDICINE

Homeopathy was discovered by Doctor Samuel Hahnemann over 200 years ago. It is a complete healing system unto itself.

At one time, there were over 150 schools of homeopathy, and it was extremely well-known throughout all of Europe and America. But at the turn of the century and the introduction of the "germ theory" and the initial fantastic results of the "silver bullets" (sulfur drugs and antibiotics), homeopathic medicine and all other types of healing (herbs, chiropractic, fasting, etc.) fell out of favor. They were ignored.

But now, after seventy years of scientific research and technological advances, we have become acutely aware of the limitations and failures of these "wonder drugs." As a result, there has been a new renaissance in the entire field of the healing arts, and one of the leaders of this new renaissance is homeopathy. Today there are thousands of doctors of homeopathy (many of whom are also medical doctors) all over the world.

Homeopathic medicine is truly the healing art for the twenty-first century because it cannot be explained by Newtonian physics. It is only with the advanced theories of Albert Einstein and Max Planck that we can begin to understand the science of homeopathy. Let me give you a few examples.

If you had a picture and cut it up in a thousand pieces and then took a few pieces away, you could never have a complete full picture again.

We also know that a minute is a minute is a minute and can never be changed in any way. How can the nature of time be altered or changed?

These statements appear true, but only if you follow the Newtonian theories of physics that we live by day to day. But these statements are not "really" true if we explore the expansive universe that we live in. One small piece of a picture can give us a perfect, exact copy of the entire picture (ever hear of a hologram?) and a minute can be a day or a second can be a year (ever hear of a black hole?). Such is the case with homeopathic medicine. It defies common logic and reason.

Through the special method and scientific procedure to prepare homeopathic medicine, it becomes *more* powerful the more you break it down. The more diluted it becomes, the more powerful it becomes. Newtonian physics cannot explain this, but with our increase of knowledge through the laws of quantum physics, homeopathy can be easily explained and understood. Maybe an example will clarify this point.

If you have a candle and you light another candle, have you taken away anything from the first candle? And if you light a thousand candles from the first original one, is the first candle lessened in any way? In fact, with one thousand candles, the light has become much more illuminating.

We usually never view medicine this way because of our constant exposure to allopathic drugs.

Allopathic drugs work on the biochemical levels of the physical body, but homeopathic medicine works on all levels on body, mind, and spirit (as some of the later stories will show). Homeopathic medicine works on what we call the "vibrational" level. It works on the vital force in the body. This force has been known throughout all of history in every civilization that has ever existed. For thousands of years, the Chinese have known it as "chi." In India, from the ancient scrolls of the ayurveda, it is known as "prana." To the Native Americans, it was revered as the "great spirit." Today, most people simply call it the "life force" within the body.

This venture into homeopathic medicine can be expounded upon in many ways, but it is not our intention to give you a history course on homeopathic medicine or a discussion on this complete, unique healing art*. What is important for you to know is that homeopathic medicine has been used safely, reliably, consistently, and effectively since its inception 200 years ago, and it has been very successful.

How successful? Let this next dramatic true personal story of an easily available over-the-counter homeopathic medicine reveal to you how incredibly dynamic and successful this medicine really is. Also remember, this one individual story is backed by millions of other successful cases from over 200 years of homeopathic medicine's history.

---

*If you want to know more about homeopathy, this intriguing 'vibrational' or 'energy' medicine for the 21st century, please go to our newsletter and read it's incredible story.

The Arnica Dragon

As I happily skipped along the stone side-walk surrounded by multicolored flowers with a deep green lawn just beyond them, I remember the hot sun high in the cloudless azure sky. The birds were singing and flying all about me, serenading me with their song. I remember thinking, "Yes, I have finally achieved my goal and reached my success. I have arrived!" My eyes soared toward the heavens with full grace and joy and happiness. I had completed my commitment of five years of school to become a doctor of chiropractic. My new clinic, The Rainbow Chiropractic Center, was open, and there were patients in the reception area waiting for my return from lunch. It was a grand and glorious day!

That was the last thing I remember. After that moment, it was all blank until I heard the clanging of metal. As I opened my eyes I was staring at the ceiling and it was moving. Confusion set in. Then I realized the ceiling wasn't moving at all, I was.

Slowly it came back to me. The pieces were falling together. Now the picture was complete. I was being pushed on a gurney down the hospital hallway with blood splattered all over me. A consuming internal survey told me I was alive with my arms and legs intact and my mind functioning properly. I was in no pain, at least at that moment. Then I went unconscious again.

My next memory was opening my eyes in the hospital bed with my girlfriend Sandra (also a doctor) holding my hand. I saw the tears in her eyes. She began to explain to me that I had been hit by a car as I was walking on the sidewalk. Her soft, gentle voice continued to assure me that everything was going to be fine.

Contrary to my last memory of no pain, my body was now in excruciating pain. I was having traumatic muscle spasms all over my body and my head was throbbing with an intense pressure. It felt like it was being crushed in a vise. I was hysterical. My mind was in a state of terror and shock. While I heard Sandra's sweet voice and felt her gentle hand I was still unable to respond. My body continued to explode in all aspects of its being.

Then in the midst of all this chaos and pain, Sandra did something very unusual—she leaned over and kissed me. It was a magical kiss that I will remember for all time. As she touched my lips, a sense of peace and tranquility came over me. An inner calm replaced my raging fear. The pain vanished. My mind was completely perplexed by what had transpired. My hysteria, my pain, my terror were gone. She drifted away, smiling. I began to speak. She responded before

I could voice the question. She said one word: "Arnica." Then I collapsed into a deep sleep.

Sleep was an endless eternity. I only know that when I opened my eyes again, Sandra was sitting by my side, whispering healing words of love and support to me. From that moment on, all was fine. Yes, there were stitches and braces and fractures, but I was going to live without any severe permanent damage.

In a few days, I was out of the hospital, much to everyone's surprise, even my own! I was amazed at my lack of pain and my spectacular recovery. Remember, I was a doctor at that time and was well aware of the normal recuperative powers of the body, and my recovery was fantastic. The doctors, nurses, everyone commented on it. I simply thanked God and never thought about it again until...

Several months later, I was in a health food store, a new one I had never been to before. As I perused the herbal remedies and the homeopathic medicines, I saw a name on one of the bottles. I did not know what it was, but it seemed familiar. My mind scanned my excellent memory banks and came up blank. Soon after, I left the store, but the name on the bottle still remained on my mind. Days went by as I continued my chiropractic clinic work. The homeopathic medicine was lingering in the back of my mind. More days went by and again I felt the shadow of a vague memory.

A few weeks later, I was at the health food store again. The name of the medicine flashed in my mind. Immediately I was on a mission quest. I marched directly to the herb and homeopathic section and grabbed the bottle that seemed to haunt me over the last few weeks and took it to the resident remedy specialist who worked there.

"Excuse me."

"Can I help you?"

"Yes, what is this? What's it for? How do you…"

Interrupting my rapid-fire questions, she responded, "It's a very powerful homeopathic remedy."

"I can see that it is a homeopathic medicine, but what's it for? What do…"

"I've never used it myself, but…"

"Then how do you know it's powerful?"

"Its success and fame are legendary."

"Really!"

"It's particularly effective for shock, trauma cases, head injuries, cuts, tears, and bruises. It is supposed to have special properties that intensifies the healing process and hastens the recovery. It's claimed to have saved people from the grip of death."

"I never heard of it."

"Well, as I said, it is very popular and very effective. It also comes as an herbal tincture, but most people use it the homeopathic form, as it appears far more helpful. Did you want this bottle?

"No, thanks, that's OK. I do not have any use for it. I'll put it back on the shelf."

I turned and walked away. Something was still unclear. Something was still echoing in my mind. Something was still playing on my head game. It would not let me rest. Then I became determined to solve the mystery. I went to the bookstore (this was before the Internet) and began my study on homeopathic medicine in general and this specific mystery homeopathic remedy. When I returned home later that night, as I came in, Sandra helped me with the groceries.

"And why art thou late, my beloved?"

"There was a dragon to slay…"

"A dragon?"

"Yes, a beastly dragon that's been pursuing me over eons of time."

"And did you render the dragon be gone and save the damsel?"

"I can assure you, my lady, 'twas no damsel in distress. Only a dragon named Arnica."

With a burst of laughter, Sandra bellowed, "The dragon Arnica? I know him well. 'Tis a powerful dragon indeed and a most benevolent one!"

"You have encountered this beast before?"

"Yes, my love, and so too, have you!"

"Me? Never have I encountered such a dragon."

"Indeed, thy memory fails thee, 'twas dragon Arnica that saved your very life."

My eyes penetrated directly into hers. "What are you saying!" I almost demanded.

"Remember when you were in the hospital and I kissed you?"

"Always I remember the magic moment, the kiss of the healing angel that calmed my heart and led me to peace."

"It was arnica that was on my lips when I kissed you and gave you the whole time you were in the hospital. That's what I said to you before you went unconscious again."

"So that's what it was! That's why when I saw the bottle of arnica homeopathic medicine at the health food store, it intrigued me. It seemed to touch some far and distant memory. I often thought about that incredible rejuvenation and recovery. It was the homeopathic medicine arnica that helped the severe head trauma and all the other injuries. It was the arnica that accelerated the entire healing process."

It was from this true personal experience that began my studies into the dynamic healing art of homeopathic medicine that eventually led me to become a Doctor of Homoeopathy.

Because of the unique nature of homeopathic medicine, do not begin to take arnica until *after* the surgery. This is when it will be most effective. Take the 12X potency, three times a day for about two weeks after the surgery, and then only once a day for another few weeks, and then discontinue. Do not take it with food or drink. Keep the bottle on hand, as it will stay potent for several years, and use it for any type of cuts or sprains or bruises or any accidents that might occur.

If you think this story is a bit exaggerated or slightly imaginative, allow me to introduce you to another incredible story told by a medical doctor in an emergency room center. This is about another type of homeopathic medicine known as the "flower remedies."*

---

* Technically, the flower remedies are not considered homeopathic medicines but for our purposes, it is not a necessary distinction

FLOWER REMEDIES

Flower remedies? I am a doctor. I work with people who are sick, who are in pain, and who are sometimes dying. I need something that works, that clears their minds, that helps their problems, that quiets their fears, that eases their pain and suffering, and that brings them to peace in their hearts. I need real medicine for people with real problems. But "flower remedies"?

For those of you not familiar with flower essences*, do not be fooled by their innocuous-sounding name. They are extremely powerful and effective remedies, as this next true life story clearly demonstrates.

---

* The term "flower remedies" and "flower essences" are interchangeable.

The Case of Dr. Michael Glazer

By its very nature, an emergency room confronts tense, critical issues and high-stress situations in every single moment. Decisions must be made in an instant. Many times, the stakes are the highest known to man—life or death.

In the blink of an eye,

in the beat of a heart,

in a thought in the mind,

in the flutter of an angel's wings,

one's life can become totally transformed.

The ambulance brought the patient in on a stretcher with oxygen and an intravenous attachment. He had suffered a massive heart attack. He was going down fast. His condition was getting worse with every moment's passing. It was only a matter of minutes, not hours but minutes, before the patient would be dead. Every possible procedure was used. He was given shots of digitalis. He was treated with electroshock therapy. He was given everything that could possibly help.

Nothing was helping.

Nothing was effective.

Nothing was slowing his descent into death.

Here was this man, in one of the most modern, sophisticated hospitals in the world, filled with all types of drugs and every technological device designed to save people's lives, but nothing was helping. This man was dying right in front of the eyes of one very helpless-feeling doctor, Dr. Michael Glazer.

The doctor did everything, absolutely everything he knew how to do, and the patient was turning blue, going into a coma, and descending deeper and deeper into death. Then it happened! By accident (if there is such a thing), in his deep despair, Dr. Glazer thrust his hands into his pockets, expressing his total frustration, his loss for anything else to do, his overwhelming sense of failure. He felt something touch the tip of his fingers. It was smooth, cold, and round.

He pulled it out of his pocket. In his left hand was a bottle, a small, insignificant bottle. It was supposed to be some New Age wonder cure-all. It was some type of homeopathic flower remedy similar to snake oil, but a modern, improved New Age version. It came to him as a gift from a friend who purchased it in a health food store. He said it was especially good for emergences, accidents, and traumas. "Why not? Nothing to lose," he thought in a curious way. He opened the bottle and gently reached out to pour a few drops of the liquid contents on the dying man's lips. It didn't even seem enough to wet them. It was only a few drops, but at that

precise time,
very instant,
exact moment,

the homeopathic medicine touched his lips, the patient's heart began to beat. His breath began to return. His date with death was interrupted. Not only was a man's life saved, a doctor's life was transformed forever. The doctor looked at the recovering patient. He looked at the label on the bottle. He looked upward toward the heavens. He looked at the bottle again. It simply said, "Homeopathic Medicine, Five Star Flower Remedy for Emergency Usage." He vowed to respect the power and validity and effectiveness and to find out all he could about these "flower remedies."

So, when people ask me about homeopathic medicine and flower remedies...

"Can they definitely make a difference?"
"Are they really effective?"
"Do they truly work?"

The answer is absolutely

Yes

Yes

Yes!

This was a dramatic, life-changing experience that transpired in a spontaneous moment, like in the previous story about the homeopathic medicine arnica.

These dynamic examples are rare, but they were selected to reveal the great healing power of homeopathic medicine. Most of the time, progress and changes are slow and gradual. The flower essences usually work in a very subtle way because they work both on the body and on the mind.

The flower essences are probably the single most important thing you can take of all the vitamins, minerals, herbs, etc., in this entire program. The reason is very simple to understand: They successfully work with our emotional states of mind. Negative states can be reduced or even eliminated, and at the same time, positive states of mind can be created. This occurs in a very slow, gentle, and subtle way, as the next story will reveal. Sometimes so subtle that you do not notice it until later when you realize, "Wow! I've been feeling really good!"

The birth of a new science known as *psychoneuroimmunology* is leading the field in researching the relationship between body, mind, and spirit, and the flower essences are at the cutting edge of this movement. They are the easiest, simplest, and safest way to prepare you emotionally for surgery. They are easily accessible from almost any health food store in the country. There are also several excellent books available that explore and explain in depth what the flower essences are, how they work, and why they are so effective. Flower remedies can have very definite effects on our emotional well-being. Somehow, flower essences can "target" different areas of our psyche or mind to create certain emotional responses in an extremely gentle way. While the mechanism for this is not clearly understood, the last fifty years of scientific testing, research studies, and clinical success have proven without a doubt that certain flower remedies can create specific emotional states. Again, I reiterate the new science of psychoneuroimmunology is validating these findings.

I've known about flower essences for years and read about the many powerful healings in which they played an essential part. In some cases, they may have been the major healing agent, but my interest was from a purely academic perspective. As stated earlier, I am a real doctor who wants, needs, and demands medicine that "really works." So, no matter how high my academic interest was, my usage was zero until one day, I meet my friend, Doctor Michael Norwood, who shared with me some of his personal and professional experiences with the flower essences. He related to me many of the clinical success stories he had with them. Then I thought, "Why not give them a try?" I did give one a try over a period of approximately a month. Nothing, absolutely nothing happened. My skepticism seemed to be justified. The flower remedy was not effective at all, so I stopped taking it. I may have been finished with the flower remedy but it was not finished with me.

The Flower Box Story

A few days later, (after I had stopped taking the flower remedy) I was walking up the front porch steps of the clinic, and the large, beautiful, red geraniums were greeting me as they did many, many times before. They were stunning. They were singing about the happiness of life. Over the twenty years at my clinic, the flowers were always colorful.

They were always a joy to my heart. Many times, I wished to sit with them and eat lunch, but the road was at this front porch, so I preferred to eat at the quieter back porch. Suddenly, an inspiration came to me. It was an idea that in all the years never came to me before. It was a simple thought, and I wondered why I never thought of it before. "Why not built a flower box on the back porch, where I usually ate lunch, so I could be surrounded by my beautiful flowers all the time? What a great idea, and it would be a matter of four pieces of wood. No special dimensions or sizes – just two long, standard-size planks and two connecting pieces. Wow! Even I could do that – make the box myself." This was not a new thought. This was a revolution. Me? Me? Me, hold a hammer in my hand – never! Ever since I became a chiropractic doctor over twenty years ago, I never held a hammer in my hand, not even to put up a picture frame. I would ask someone or pay someone to do the job, but me bang a nail—never!

I am not proud about this, but my hands were and are sacred to me, and I never use them for manual labor – not to hammer a nail, not to cut a piece of wood, paint a wall, push a lawn mower, wash dishes, shovel snow, bag leaves, change a flat tire – nothing. You will understand why I am so adamant on making this point when you read the dialogue between Dr. Michael Norwood and myself sometime afterwards.

"Louis, how have you been?"

"Super as always."

"Are you enjoying the conference?"

"Yes, it always feels good to learn more."

"By the way, did you ever get around to using those 'flower remedies' like you said you were?"

"Yes, Michael, I did."

"And?"

"Nothing."

"You're not serious?"

"Nothing."

"They were and are very effective for me and for my patients all the time," Dr. Michael insisted.

"Well, I am very glad they work for you and your patients, but they didn't do anything for me. Case closed. But I will tell you the big news."

"You have my full attention."

"I built a flower box for the back porch."

"No way! Who helped?"

"No one, really, all by myself!"

"I do not believe it – YOU?" He was laughing as he said this.

"I'm telling you: I went down to the lumber store and spoke with the man. It was so funny! He was asking me about the dimensions, what type of wood, what size nails, etc.

"I need some wood for a flower box outside," I tell him.

"You want something treated then."

"Treated for what?"

"For outside—the rain, termites, things that determine the integrity of the structure and its longevity."

"Well, I guess, if you say so."

"What size?"

"I don't know – what's a standard stock size?"

"Eight feet, ten feet, and twelve feet."

"I guess twelve feet would be fine."

"How deep do you want the flower bed?"

"I don't know; how wide is the wood?"

"Six inches, eight inches, and ten inches."

"I'll take the ten-inch."

"So, this goes on for about twenty five minutes where the guy is asking me all these questions and he's laughing at me the whole time because he realizes I have no clue to what I'm doing and just making it up as we go along. Finally, I get all the wood, pick the nails, and then he tells me I can rent a hammer and any other equipment instead of buying it. Michael, before you know it, I'm at the clinic, and I'm pounding and sawing and sweating and working, and I'm feeling great. I'm loving it! Now I'm on a roll, so for the next five days straight, I'm back at the lumber yard, buying stuff. I'm renting drills and post-hole diggers, and electric saws – everything! I'm digging holes, I fixed the fence, put new doors on the storage shed, put in a new mailbox. I'm doing it."

Dr. Norwood was astonished! "Not possible – Doctor Louis Leonardi did this?"

"All by myself," I asserted proudly.

"Everything?" he asked with big, bewildered eyes, not believing a word.

"All the measuring, hammering, cutting, digging – EVERYTHING! I even put the soil in the flower box and planted the flowers."

"Wow, this is an incredible story!" Dr. Michael finally conceded with a little smirk on his face.

The conference was about to begin again, so we turned to go inside. As an afterthought, Dr.

Michael said, "Louis, by the way, what flower remedy did you use?"

"I used the one for..."

The veil lifted from my eyes. "Michael, Michael, I can't believe it! It can't be! I can't believe the implication!"

"What are you talking about—the flower remedy?"

"Yes, Michael, I took the flower remedy for 'strength'!"

He looked at me in full awareness and understanding of what had transpired. Then he said, "What type of strength are you talking about—inner strength like fortitude or courage or...?"

"No, Michael that's the point. I was thinking about pure and raw muscular strength. That's what the desire was in my mind at the moment. I took that specific remedy because that's what I wanted – physical power."

Dr. Michael responded, "What did you imagine, a few drops on the tongue every day would turn you into Hercules?"

"I don't know. I simply thought about being stronger, physically in my body."

"Lifting wood and sawing boards and pounding nails would build muscle. Maybe it was just a coincidence," he laughed as he looked me in the eyes and said, "Strength...and you told me the flower remedy did not work!"

It was an incredible revelation for me, and yes, I can admit that it was a coincidence except for one thing—over the last dozen years, the flower remedies have been very effective and successful! I have used them for myself and hundreds of my patients with great success. Believe me! These flower remedies truly are fantastic and will help you tremendously. They can affect many of the emotional states of mind that we experience on a day-to-day basis. Feelings like low self-esteem, lack of confidence, self-doubt, rage, jealousy, depression, excessive pride, and many others, can all be affected with the use of the flower remedies. In fact, the flower remedies can help us not only eliminate these emotional states but can create positive ones like confidence, tranquility, joy, and even love. Thirty-eight emotional states have been established with a definite flower for each of these states.

With this basic background, let us examine the flower remedies that would be best for you.

After working in a surgical center, it became apparent through my own observations and in speaking with patients, that people underwent three consistent basic emotional challenges: worry, anxiety, and fear. To help us reduce and overcome these emotional challenges, the following suggestions are made:

Condition	*Suggested Flower Remedy*
Worry	Agrimony
Anxiety	Rock Rose
Fear	Mimulus

These are the names of the individual flower essences. They are usually available at any good health food store.

Put equal amounts of all three remedies in a small bottle and take a few drops three times a day, every day, until the day before the event. Put the drops directly on the tongue and do not mix with anything. It is best taken alone and not with meals. You can drink water immediately after if you wish.* These three flower remedies are known to be of great benefit in relieving these negative states of mind and producing much more positive ones. They will replace worry with understanding, anxiety with peace, and fear with wisdom and courage.

---

* The flower remedies are in an alcohol base, so if that is a consideration, then place a few drops in a cup of boiling water, then let the water cool down, then drink the water. The heat will evaporate the alcohol.

One Week Before

Surgery is a week away. Continue to relax. Remember the most important information is found in Part I of this book. Read it again

slowly,

carefully,

completely.

It will make all the difference in the world.

We will add no other suggestions or recommendations at this time except one: begin to take "bromelain." It is a supplement that will keep the inflammatory response to a complete minimum. Take it at three times the recommended dosage. You might also like to drink some pineapple juice, which contains large amounts of bromelain, but get *real* pineapple juice not "pineapple drink," because the drinks usually contain large amounts of sugar, which you are trying to avoid.

Every other part of the *pre surgical care* program should remain constant unless the doctor tells you otherwise. In fact, be sure to continue to follow your doctor's advice first and foremost throughout this entire program.

Diet:	remains the same
Fresh Juicing:	remains the same
Exercise:	remains the same
Vitamins:	remains the same
Minerals:	remains the same
Herbs:	remains the same
Homeopathic:	remains the same
Flower Remedies:	remains the same

All these are to remain the same, except adding the bromelain as just noted. It is not necessary to do every single aspect of this program. Just follow it easily, willingly, playfully. It is far more important and beneficial to simply read this book and stay relaxed and stress-free.

One Day Before

Today is the day before surgery. Great! You did it! You accepted your challenge. You achieved your goal. You fulfilled your commitment. Give yourself all congratulations. Give yourself total acknowledgment. Give yourself full credit. This is what you have worked for all these many days. You've done your best, and you have prepared well. You're ready to complete this task and move on with your life. Now, relax with a job well done.

Forget all the vitamins, minerals, and supplements. Forget everything—absolutely everything. Take a deep breath and relax.

No matter how much or little you have done, remember the inspiring words of Bob Wieland: "Last? Never!"

Sometimes in the course of this book, I may have seemed overly dramatic or exaggerating the concerns of your individual situation. If so, please forgive me.

But if your surgery is of a serious nature, then please allow me to say this—no one knows the path or destiny of another. No matter what you have been told or how unfavorable it may appear, know this in all aspects of your being...

Where there is Life

There is Always

Hope

In the known and unknown universe, throughout the eons of time and timelessness, in the infinity of existence, there is no force, no energy, nothing that is greater than the

Power

of

Prayer

Read these words over and over and over and over again and again and again. Let these words linger in your mind. Let them meander into your cells. Let them radiate throughout your spirit. Let them sink deep into your soul, then please follow this one suggestion—take time to reflect, create a moment of silence, and then pray. Again, I say to you, take time to reflect, create a moment of silence, and pray.

Give thanks, give praise, and give blessing for this opportunity that you have been given for this surgery. Say thanks to everyone in the hospital or clinic tomorrow. Tell everyone how grateful you are for their help and the kindness they have shown you and are showing you now. Let them experience your inner strength, your peace, your tranquility, your humor, and your smile. Make their day a little lighter, a little easier. With this attitude, all around you will be full of love, joy, and grace!

In this way, with these vibrations surrounding you, there could be only one outcome. Know, with a full, absolute knowing, that there can be only one true outcome, and it can be expressed in one word—

Divine

Epilogue

The surgery is over. All is well. Rejoice and celebrate. Give thanks, praise, and blessings. Return to the *pre surgical care* program and continue on it for the next month with the exception of the flower remedies. Stop taking them and begin taking the homeopathic medicine arnica as indicated earlier. Now engage your mind's powerful healing abilities to begin your complete and total accelerated regeneration and rejuvenation and recuperation. You can begin the healing process with a sound. Research has clearly shown this sound is always associated with positive and joyous emotions. This sound has a profound affect on our hormonal system, metabolic system, and immune system. In fact, not just every system in our body but every single cell in our body will perform better. It also has a great impact on our emotional well-being. It will be a very wonderful, positive, and effective way to begin the healing process.

The well-known author Norman Cousins, in his best-selling book, *Anatomy of an Illness*, credits this sound with healing him of his so-called terminal cancer. It is a sound that you can create. Yes, you can do it. Let it be a sign of your courage and acceptance, a symbol of the joy in your heart, and example of your love and inspiration. Yes, you can do it. You can create this sound in this wonderful moment.

It is

the most beautiful sound,

the most profound sound,

the most inspirational sound,

the most joyous sound that ever touched the earth
and spread throughout the universe.

The sound? The sound is the sound of…

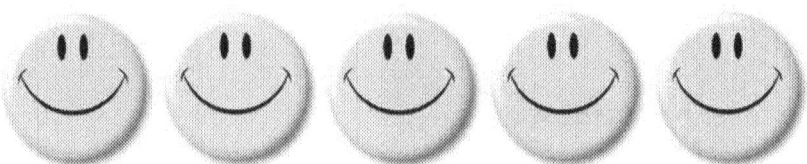

Laughter

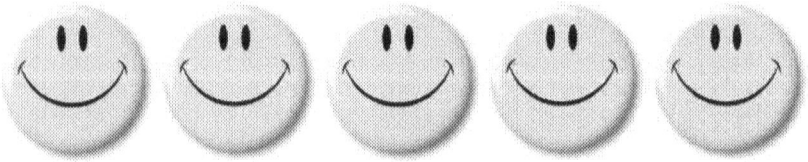

Laughter

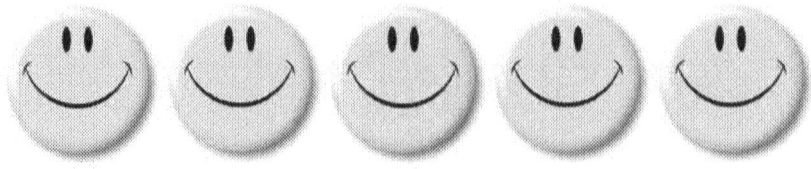

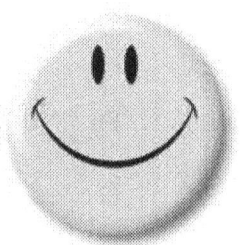

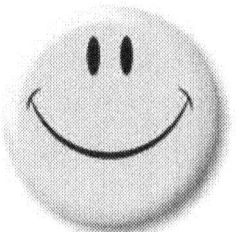

As you continue to move forward with your wonderful smile and life, please consider this:

Give this book to someone else you know, please. Don't let it just sit on a shelf. Surely there is someone you know and love who would benefit from reading this book and following this program.

Give it to your surgeon. Suggest he give it to other surgeons or other patients. Pre Surgical Care *is for everyone.*

Give it to a stranger. Let them know there is still hope, and caring, and love in the world.

Dannion Brinkley wrote a true international best-selling book *Saved by the Light*, which was later the inspiration for a special television movie. It was about his near-death experience. He said he reviewed his life from "the other side," and he saw all the things he had ever done. He saw everything throughout his entire life. In his review, he saw one of the single, most wonderful things he ever did—a valued lesson, a highlight in his life, a great moment—was when he gave a sandwich to a hungry man!

It was a simple act of kindness. Maybe, just maybe, your giving this book to someone else will be remembered as a great act of kindness.

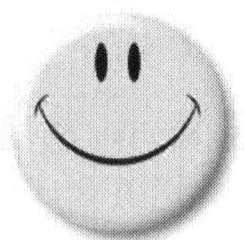

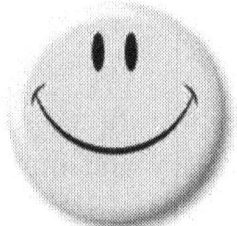

Pre Surgical Care Gift Program

There is one unique way that always succeeds in letting someone know they are very special—it is giving them a gift.

The Pre Surgical Care Gift Program is designed for that purpose and much more. Not only are you letting that person know you care and are thinking about them, but you will also be sending them something that can truly benefit their life.
It will be a gift to help support them in this time of trepidation, from a tooth extraction to a cancerous tumor—from stitches to micro skin grafts—from a facelift to heart surgery. This book will be a gift that will tell them that you are with them.

It will be a wonderful gift—a gift that will give them not only useful, necessary and important information to help ensure they have a safe, simple, and successful surgery, but also a gift that will tell them they are not alone.

A gift that will be full of

care and concern,

purpose and meaning,

support and love.

It will be a gift that they will always remember and appreciate.

We can send a beautifully gift-wrapped special hardcover edition of *Pre Surgical Care*, signed by the author, including your own personal message to anyone, anywhere in the world.

Pre Surgical Care Gift Order Form

A special hardcover edition of **Pre Surgical Care** will be signed by the author and beautifully gift-wrapped. It will include your personal message and delivered to anyone, anywhere in the world.

To: Name _____

Address _____

_____

City_____State_____Zip_____

From: Name _____

Address _____

_____

City_____State_____Zip_____

Your personal message to be included: _____

_____

_____

_____

_____

_____

_____

_____

Form of payment: _____ personal check _____ money order

Credit Card number: _____ expiration date_____
(Visa/MasterCard)

Signature _____

Please send $22.50   plus $9.95 (shipping & gift wrapping) total $32.45
                                $30.77 (international)   total $53.27

Send to: Pre Surgical Care
                1358 Hawthorne Ave.
                Smyrna, GA 30080
                U.S.A.

Email: drleonardi@presurgicalcare.com

Website: www.presurgicalcare.com

Newsletter: www.presurgicalcare.com

Phone/Fax: (770) 434-8310

Skype: (267) 828-0125

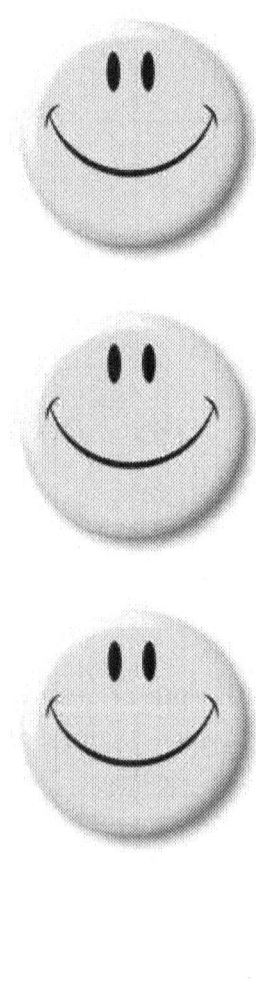
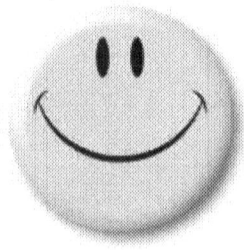

Post Surgical Care

As mentioned earlier in this book, we suggest you continue on the Pre Surgical Care program for the month after the surgery, with the exception of the flower remedies, which will be stopped and replaced with the homeopathic medicine arnica. There are also additional steps that can be taken that will help the process of a complete recuperation, regeneration, and rejuvenation. These will be suggestions like probiotics, enzymes, tissue salts, and more.

We are preparing this important information into a forthcoming book that will be called *Post Surgical Care*. It will be published as soon as possible, but since it is not available yet, we have decided to publish a newsletter that will give you this vital information as it is being developed, plus other ideas and tips on health and healing.

This is a free service to you and anyone else. Everyone will benefit from this information. Please e-mail us and get on our mailing list so we can give you the latest and best advice possible for the quickest recovery, regeneration, and rejuvenation possible, and other advice on health and healing. Please, if you have any questions on health and healing, do not hesitate to contact us. Remember we cannot diagnose or prescribe or suggest any course of action. We can give you information only for educational purposes, which we will be very glad to do. If we can be of service to you, please contact us.

DrLeonardi@PreSurgicalCare.com

Or leave a message at: 770-434-8310

You can also go to our Web site, which will give you additional helpful information.

www.PreSurgicalCare.com

The Pre Surgical Care Internet Journal

The Pre Surgical Care Internet Journal Newsletter is wide ranging and comprehensive. It is free to anyone and everyone all over the world. It is a source for information that is non commercial, unbiased, educational, interesting, and most importantly practical and useful. As a true newsletter should be, it is not an advertising commercial, it is a service.

We sell nothing. We endorse nothing. We promote nothing except vibrant health a dynamic, positive mental attitude and an uplifting and joyous spirit.

The Pre Surgical Care Internet Journal Newsletter gives you information on all the latest developments in pre and post surgical care, research breakthroughs, technological advances plus an extensive range of topics in the healing arts. You will receive articles and feature stories written by many different types of doctors not only in the field of allopathic medicine like orthopedic surgeons, neurologist, dentists, ophthalmologists, etc. but also doctors from the holistic area of the healing arts.

Doctors of naturopathy will share with you their knowledge about herbs and possible alternatives for allopathic drugs. They can also help you with information on nutrition, diet, exercise and many other things.

Doctors of homeopathy will give you an in depth understanding of this unique healing system. They will share with you various homeopathic medicines that are beneficial for particular problems.

Acupuncturists will speak to you about "energy medicine" and what they accomplish beyond just "sticking, you with needles".

And doctors of chiropractic will help you to understand that through the use of manipulations and its effect on the nervous system they can help alleviate a wide range of health problems.

You will be given information about little known but very effective treatments like:

- enzymes --- necessary for proper digestion
- flower remedies --- that can improve your emotional well being
- cranial manipulations --- that have been successful in healing certain cases of epilepsy
- probiotics --- essential bacteria in your intestinal tract that must be replaced after any use of antibiotics
- tissue salts --- necessary ultra-molecular minerals that can balance your blood
- applied kinesiology --- a simple diagnostic technique that can find neurological problems like dyslexia and other learning disabilities, especially in children
- aromatherapy --- an easy way to cleanse and purify the air in your home and create a healthy and peaceful environment
- scar removal massage--- a way to reduce and possibly totally eliminate scars from your surgery or other scars that you were told were permanent and unchangeable, even if these scars are years old.

These are only some of the many topics that you will learn about and be able to use that will benefit your health. In fact, our newsletter is so extensive that, with your interest and participation, we have set up a program that will allow you to receive a certificate of diplomat and possibly even a doctorate if you fulfill all the necessary requirements. Otherwise just relax, read it and enjoy!

All this is available through the use of the Pre Surgical Care Internet Journal Newsletter and there is even one more very special feature that we feel is the greatest service of all ----- the ability for you to ask us your questions and get real, direct, straightforward answers. This is virtually unprecedented in the field of newsletters on the internet and anywhere else. As a part of subscribing to our free newsletter you will have the ability to ask your myriad of questions and have an interactive relation with us and all the various doctors and professionals that we are associated with. In the near future you will be able to speak to Dr. Leonardi and all the experts he works with directly as he will be hosting his own internet show.

We are also giving away a music CD designed especially for healing. For more information on this extra bonus go to the next chapter on the special incentive offer award and get the details so you can receive this free gift.

Even if you do not buy the Pre Surgical Care book, copy down our internet newsletter address and you can download this very special healing music for free. Subscribe to our free newsletter now and begin to enjoy this excellent newsletter today.

www.PreSurgicalCare.com

Its all free.

Its all available.

Its all waiting for you.

Thank you.

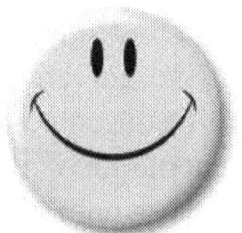

THE SPECIAL INCENTIVE
OFFER AWARD

The Special Incentive Offer Award of the healing music that is available here is very simple and easy to obtain.

Why the healing music?

Throughout all of ancient history, from the rhythmic drumming in the primitive wilds of Africa to the advanced civilizations on the River of the Nile, music has been sacred and used in ceremony and healing. It has been only in the last few centuries that the universal role of music as an effective healing agent has been eclipsed to become used merely for entertainment purposes. But the ability of music to heal is as powerful and dynamic today as ever.

As we learn more and more about the energies, the vibrations, the electromagnetic fields of this wondrous universe we come to realize that it is these forces that serve as the patterns, the codes, the predecessors, the blue prints for every biological being on the planet, from the smallest virus, to the petals of the rose, to the great whales of the deep, to every single cell of the human body. All are the result of these electromagnetic fields. These forces do not radiate from the physical, in essence they create the physical.

The biochemical, mechanistic view of the body, which is still taught in every medical school in the country, is an old, outdated and antiquated model that absolutely does not work. It completely neglects the electromagnetic energies that permeate the entire body and exist throughout the deepest depths of space.

In his ground breaking study for "Nature", a preeminent scientific journal, the renowned biophysics F. Weinholt tells us *"conventional medical researchers have no understanding of the molecular mechanisms that truly provide for life"*.

Dr. Bruce Lipton in his revolutionary, best selling book "The Biology of Belief", reveals to us, in no uncertain terms, how the Newtonian laws of physics, which is the main stay of the whole of modern medicine, is a mechanical model which does not and cannot explain any of the biological processes of the human body. It is only though quantum physics that these processes can be explained. He continues to point out to us *"hundreds upon hundreds of scientific research studies over the last fifty years have consistently revealed that invisible forces of the electromagnetic spectrum profoundly impact every facet of biological regulation. These energies include... acoustic frequencies. Specific frequencies and patterns of electromagnetic radiation regulate DNA, RNA, and protein syntheses, alter protein shape and function, and control gene regulation, cell division, cell differentiation, morphogenesis (the process by which cells assemble into organs and tissues), hormone secretion, nerve growth and function."*

If you can truly understand what is being explicitly stated, you can clearly see the incredible impact that certain vibrations, energies, frequencies, created from the pluck of a string, hence music, can alter and change and enhance our entire being of body, mind and spirit.

Remember, at the correct intensity and frequency, the human voice can shatter glass.

The offer of this healing music that we make to you here is not of a trite nature. This music was sincerely and specifically designed for your use during the surgery and while it will help you to relax and become peaceful at anytime it goes far beyond that. It possesses a tremendous healing force that will have an uplifting, regenerating, and rejuvenating effect on all levels of your body, mind and spirit.

If you want to know more about how this particular healing music came about, read the newsletter to discover this fantastic true story.

This exquisite healing music will be wonderful to use with the mental techniques for visualization, affirmations, and being in the silence or any time you wish to become relaxed and peaceful.

It is also intended to be used during the surgery itself. Simply get a small personal CD player with earphones and listen to this healing music during the surgery itself. It is doubtful that your doctor will have much of an idea of all that has been written about in this chapter about the powerful effects that this music will have on you but he should have no objection in allowing you to do this.

Purchase the book, fill out and send us the original form (no copies please, it must be the original form) and receive this music CD designed specifically for healing.

That's it. No shipping charges. No mailing cost. No handling fee. Nothing. It's that simple. Done!

Subscribe to our newsletter, which is also free, and you will receive the specially designed music for healing. Just send us your e-mail address so we can send you our newsletter and download to you this truly enlightening music. That's it. Done!

Please note again that this incentive award for the CD is offered on a limited basis. Please act now so you do not miss out on this excellent opportunity.

As for the healing music itself, it will always be available as a download from our website and the Pre Surgical Care Internet Journal Newsletter.

Make copies and/or forward it to your friends, family and loved ones. Maybe even your not so friends or not so loved ones. Maybe it will surprise them and touch them in an unknown beautiful way.

This too would be a "simple act of kindness".

Thank you.

Simply fill out this form completely and send it along (remove this page from the book) to the address below to receive your free special healing music CD:

Name:

Street:

City:

State:

Zip:

Country:

Email address:

Phone:

Send to:
Pre Surgical Care
1358 Hawthorne Ave
Smyrna, GA 30080
USA

Note: only this original page that has been removed from the book will be accepted.

The Third Option

This entire book has always been

    optimistic

        practical

            energetic

                supportive

                    positive

                        uplifting

                            empowering

                            and hopefully inspiring

Let us continue in this same vein but if you still have fears and concerns and doubts allow me to present to you this website and read all about another possibility:

www.thethirdoption.org

www.infinityhealingarts.com

Resources
Obtaining Products

A good way to proceed with the supplement part of this program is to:

1. Go to the health food store and buy everything at once. Anything you cannot find at the health food store ask them if they can special order it or advise you about it.
2. Another easy way to obtain all the items in the Pre Surgical Care program is to go to www. HealingArtsFulfillment.com They are a fulfillment company that has been created to make it extremely easy for you to obtain all the necessary products for the Pre Surgical Care program. With one single contact through:

   • e-mail info@healingartsfulfillment.com

   • fax 267-7506919

   • telephone 267- 750-6919

   • website www.HealingArtsFulfillment.com

You can order the complete package of everything you need, even the laughter.

You must specify to them the herbs that you have selected so they can be properly added. Also be sure to order by authors name, Dr. Louis Leonardi, and book title "Pre Surgical Care". It's that simple, one contact and you have the complete Pre Surgical Care program in one single box.

Because of the nature of a fulfillment company please do not request them to send out only certain items. It is a complete package ready to be sent to you.

Please note. Even though these supplements are not prescription items some of them are available only through doctors. Therefore these professional products that will be sent to you are of an extremely high quality and may cost slightly more than what you would find in health food stores and on the internet. It would appear that under the circumstances these higher costs would be acceptable and the ensured benefits justifiable. But as this program has stated many times, the choice is yours---always.

Use this summary list to assist you in obtaining what you want. Bring it to the health food store and check things off as you get them. Make a special note of the things that you need for a two-month supply. This will be for the post-surgical care.

<u>Summary list</u>

Vitamin A, C, and E

Multi-mineral formula

Zinc

Manganese

Herbs_____

Homeopathic Medicine – Arnica (12X)

Flower Remedy - Agrimony

Flower Remedy - Rock Rose

Flower Remedy - Mimulus

One new dropper bottle to mix the flower remedies

Laughter   Laughter   Laughter

Whole Foods Market
550 Bowie Street
Austin, TX 78703
512-477-4455
voicemail 512-477-5566
fax 512-482-7000
www. wholefoodsmarket. com

Trace Mineral Research
P.O. Box 429
Roy, Utah 84067
www.traceminerals.com

Nutri-West
P.O. Box 23004
Hilton Head, South Carolina 29925
800-334-3793 or 843-342-3688
www.nutriwestblueridge.com

Standard Process Inc.
1200 West Royal Lee Drive
Palmyra, Wisconsin 53149
www.standardprocess.com

A.C. Grace Company
1100 Quitman Drive
P.O. Box 570
Sandy Plains, Texas 75755
800-833-4368
903-636-4368
www.acgraceco.com

Biotics Research Corp
6801 Biotics Research Drive
Rosenburg, Texas 77471
800-231-5777
fax 281-344-0725
www.bioticresearch.com

Herbs of Light Inc.
P.O. Box 1648
High Springs, Florida 32655
800 313-3011
fax 800-837-2244
www.herbsoflight.com
info@herbsoflight.com

Eclectic Institute Inc.
14385 SE Lusted Road
Sandy, Oregon 97005
800-332-4372
www.eclecticherb.com

Herb-Farm
P.O. Box 116
Williams, Oregon 97544
800-348-4372
www.herb-pharm.com
info@herb-pharm.com

Herbs Etc., Inc.
1345 Cerrillos Road
Santa Fe, New Mexico 87505
888-694-3727
fax 888-437-2738
www.herbsetc.com

Boiron
Campus Blvd
Building A
Newton Square, Pennsylvania 19073
800-blue-tube
610-325-7464

Newton Laboratories Inc.
2360 Rockaway Industrial Blvd.
Conyers, Georgia 30012
800-448-7256
fax 770-388-7768
www.newtonlabs.net
info@newtonlabs.net

Flower Essence Services
P.O. Box 1769
Nevada City, California 95959
800-548-0075
fax 530-265-6467
www.fesflowers.com
info@fesflowers.com

Dr. Edward Bach Center
Mount Vernon Bakers Lane
Sotwell, Oxon OX10 OPZ
United Kingdom
44-1491-834-678
www.bachcentre.com

ACKNOWLEDGMENTS

To Wayne in Barbados, who was with me when the book began, and listened to me and allowed me to tell him all my ideas—I say thank you.

To Heather, my Bali angel, who transcribed the first page from my hand-scribbled notes—I say thank you.

To Barbara, who organized and completed the first draft and brought the book into physical manifestation and continued to help and support me every step of the way—I say thank you.

A Martial qui a transforme cette mouture en phase finale electronique—je dis merci.

To Richard Carter, the artist, who helped me create this beautiful cover—I say thank you.

To AuthorHouse, for the publication of my book—I say thank you

To Bruce Briscoe, whose excitement and enthusiasm and computer expertise helped me to spread this message all over the world—I say thank you.

To Dr. Martin Finkelestein. who is always supporting and encouraging me to be the best I could be—I say thank you.

To Dr. Michael Norwood, for all his support and the technical assistance that he always was so generous in giving to me—I say thank you.

To Carter Liu, the computer genius who always assisted me with my questions—I say thank you.

To Dr. David Schneider, who gave me hope for the book's success—I say thank you.

To Dr. Alannah Levian, for her vast knowledge of the healing arts and sharing that knowledge with me over many years—I say with all love, thank you.

To Richard Katz and Patricia Kaminski who have always been so giving to me with their wisdom of the flower essences—I say thank you.

Vielen Dank An Helmut Maier der mich immer mit seinen schonen fotografien von blumen inspiriert hat.

To Stacy Robyn my unknown friend—I say Go Gratitude.

To Dr. Lou Da Trinco, who kept me alive to be able to complete the book—I can never say thank you enough.

Dan yang paling penting adalah untuk kekasihku tersayang Safna yang dengan setia duduk disampingku hari demi hari ketika aku menulis buku ini—Terima kasih.

To all my friends and family who have given me their talents and support and love to make my life so joyously happy—I say thank you and thank you and thank you.

To Starlord—always.

To Kistay—with love.

To Lord Ginga—all grace.

To the fire of Agnihotra—forever.

To Sumiyati – temanku.

To the Wind that carries my most beloved friends the Golden Eagle, the Mighty Sparrow, and the Great Condor—let us fly together forever.

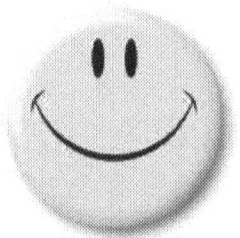

Author

After a remarkably successful academic and athletic career at New York University, Louis Leonardi graduated and went on to become a doctor. He became involved with all aspects of the healing arts. During the last twenty-five years, he has been involved with both research and clinical practice. Beyond his formal academic studies, his quest for knowledge in the healing arts has taken him to the far corners of the world. Doctor Leonardi has studied herbs and natural remedies with the shaman in the rainforests of Central and South America. He has gone to Africa to study the ways of the traditional tribal medicine men. He has worked with acupuncturists in Indonesia and China. Doctor Leonardi has also studied with the doctors of ayurvedic medicine and homeopathy in India.

His career has included being a team doctor at the Olympic Games, working with celebrities and global leaders, and taking care of the homeless and needy. He has given care to indigenous people all over the world through the four free clinics he has established on three continents.

Doctor Leonardi has appeared on radio and television all over the world. He has published many articles for magazines and newspapers, as well as presented papers at scientific congresses both nationally and internationally.

He is eager to share, and hopes that it inspires others, to know that if a former New York City taxicab driver can go on to do these things, anybody can!

www.ingramcontent.com/pod-product-compliance
Lightning Source LLC
Chambersburg PA
CBHW032023170526
45157CB00002B/839